Custom LASIK

Presented by

R.K. Ghosheh, MD
Faris R. Ghosheh, MD

United States Copyright 2008
Published by MWP Media
Cover designed by Han Le
ISBN 13: 978-0-9818209-0-3
ISBN 10: 0-9818209-0-5

Disclaimer

The information presented in this book is not intended to replace medical advice of your personal physician or any surgeon performing LASIK surgery. In addition, the information expressed by authors in this book is the opinion of the authors based on experience in performing laser vision correction.

Table of Contents

Chapter **Page**

Introduction iv

1 *Custom LASIK* 1

2 *Eye Anatomy and Function* 4

3 *Refractive Error* 9

4 *Refractive Surgical Procedures* 23

5 *LASIK and the New Advancements* 29

6 *Wavefront* 36

7 *Selecting the Right LASIK Surgeon* 46

8 *Initial Consultation* 58

9 *The Day of Your Custom LASIK Procedure* 67

10 *Postoperative Care after Custom LASIK* 73

11 *Patient Results from Custom LASIK* 78

12 *Possible Risks with Custom LASIK* 82

13 *Questions and Answers* 89

Conclusion 94

Appendix *History—Timeline of Refractive Surgery* 95

Introduction

AT THE ANNUAL MEETING OF THE American Society of Cataract and Refractive Surgery (ASCRS) an independent researcher and eye surgeon reported that "Custom LASIK produces superior vision quality compared to traditional LASIK eye surgery."

He indicated that while conventional LASIK is satisfactory, Custom LASIK "yields sharper and higher quality vision, and higher patient satisfaction compared to conventional LASIK. The improvement will likely be most apparent when driving at night," said US Navy Captain Steve Schallhorn, MD, the Director of Cornea and Refractive Surgery at the Navy Medical Center, San Diego.

This surgeon went on to explain that custom LASIK, performed on Navy and Marine Corps personnel, had improved the quality of vision resulting in fewer halos and glare.

The presenter showed that of the patients who underwent conventional LASIK, 88 percent achieved 20/20 or better after six months. While patients who underwent Custom LASIK, 97 percent achieved 20/20 or better. Better still, 85 percent of patients having Custom LASIK achieved 20/16, compared to 69 percent of patients who achieved 20/16 with conventional LASIK.

These are startling findings when you compare the disparity between conventional LASIK and Custom LASIK which offers superior vision for many.

So, what is Custom LASIK? Is this eye surgery really safe? How long has it been around? How do you know if you are a good candidate? Who should perform the surgery? This book is designed to help you answer all of these questions.

1
Custom LASIK

Custom LASIK is the most advanced vision correction system that blends surgical skill with complex technology to treat both large and small imperfections in vision, helping patients see well both day and night.

The first step is the surgical consultation. The surgeon evaluates your prescription, corneal thickness, corneal map, pupil size, tear film, cornea, and lens. In some patients, more advanced mapping of the vision system is performed, called the wavefront map. The surgeon then determines what type of vision correction procedure is best for you. Is it LASIK? PRK? LASEK? Lens surgery? Intacs? Or are you better off staying with your glasses and contacts?

For most patients, LASIK is the best option. The surgeon then determines how long you will need to be out of contact lenses. This can range from one week to several months, depending on the shape of your cornea. After you've been out of contact lenses for the recommended amount of time, your pre-procedural measurements are performed.

The surgeon then creates a treatment plan based on your unique vision needs and anatomy. Part of this plan is customizing the first step of the LASIK procedure – creation of the superficial corneal layer, also called the flap that will then be lifted to access the inner corneal layers. With conventional LASIK, a surgical blade is used to form the flap. But with advances in technology, we no longer need to do that. We can now use the precision of a unique laser system, called Intralase femtosecond laser, to safely and accurately create the flap. Moreover, we can customize this step to fit each patient's individual anatomy. Do you have smaller eyes? Do you have thinner corneas? These factors could have prevented you from getting LASIK in the past. Not anymore. With the customized first step, we can proceed with LASIK in many patients who couldn't have it in the past.

After the first procedure step is completed, the surgeon reshapes your inner cornea to correct your nearsightedness, farsightedness, and/or astigmatism as well as smaller imperfections in vision to give you good day and night vision. The corneal reshaping is often based on the wavefront map of your vision.

During the wavefront mapping, the light is sent into the eye in a specific pattern, and then measured after it has passed through the visual system. Any differences between what goes in and what is measured is considered an aberration. Think of a square grid going in and a wavy grid coming out. The waves represent aberrations. These aberrations are both the larger imperfections in your vision, such as myopia, hyperopia and astigmatism, as well as smaller imperfections in your vision, such as spherical aberration, coma, and trefoil. Larger imperfections are called lower order aberrations (LOA) and smaller imperfections are called higher order aberrations (HOA).

A common eye examination and refraction evaluates only LOA. Your glasses and contacts correct only LOA. You need them corrected to see well enough to function in your daily activities. You may, however, have noticed that night driving can be difficult sometimes even with glasses and contacts. You may have glare, halos, or simply difficulty discerning objects in dim light. The reason here is that your HOA are not corrected.

Only a wavefront map is able to measure HOA. Wavefront technology as a diagnostic device is unsurpassed.

With this technology, the surgeon can diagnose and measure aberrations that no other system can detect. It is important to understand that without a wavefront diagnosis, it is impossible for a surgeon to accurately determine if wavefront-guided correction is necessary for a good LASIK, PRK, or LASEK outcome. Conversely, without a wavefront diagnosis it is impossible for a surgeon to accurately determine if a wavefront ablation is not necessary. In other words, virtually every person considering laser vision correction should have a wavefront diagnostic evaluation.

With the wavefront eye examination the surgeon creates a "map" of vision imperfections. A conventional eye exam maps refraction and evaluates lower order aberrations. A wavefront diagnostic, however, maps both lower order aberrations and high order aberrations.

The pattern of imperfections or the wavefront map is unique to each patient. This map is electronically transferred into the excimer laser which the surgeon will then apply to reshape your vision.

There are unique challenges for application of the wavefront technology. The human eye is not static as with a telescope; it offers dynamic movements and alternating normal biological functions such as focus and pupil size. It therefore requires skill on the part of the surgeon to analyze all the features unique to your vision and synthesize a treatment strategy to correct your vision safely and accurately.

With Custom LASIK, we are at the forefront of the safest, most accurate methods for corrected vision. However, the procedure is not for everyone. It is for this reason that you should know as much as possible about what Custom LASIK is and whether or not you should have it done.

2

Eye Anatomy and Function

IF YOU UNDERSTAND how the eye works, you will understand refractive surgery. The primary purpose of your eye is to focus, or refract light. When the rays of light are not focused or refracted properly, you need glasses, contact lenses, or surgery to correct this condition.

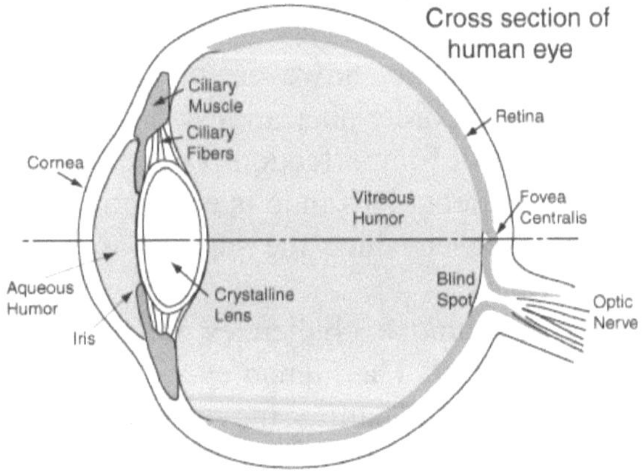

The Human Eye

Your eye works very much like a camera. Light enters the eye through the cornea – the clear front surface or the "window" of the eye. As the light passes through the cornea, it is bent or refracted. This bent light then travels through the pupil and into the lens. The lens acts to fine tune the focus of light onto the retina. The retina turns the light energy into electrical impulses that travel along the optic nerve from the eye to the brain, where the image is interpreted.

Notice the illustrations depict various parts of the eye that will help you understand the vision process and why vision can be distorted.

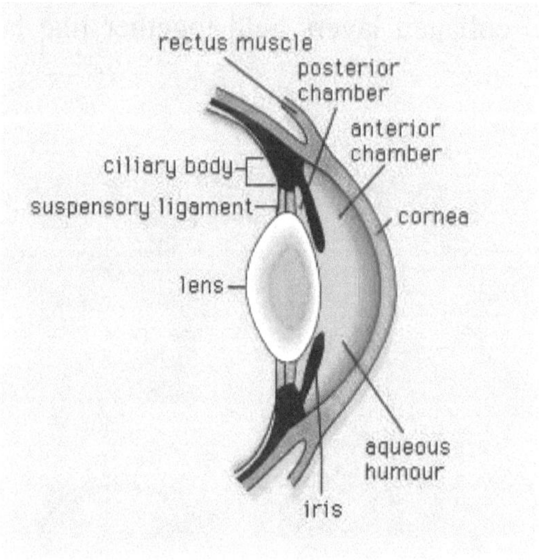

Parts of the Human Eye

Sclera

The sclera is the support layer of the eye. It is the white part of the eye that you see in the mirror and it provides structure and protection for the cornea.

Cornea

The cornea is the front-most surface of the eye and provides most of the eye's focusing power. Most of the refracting (bending) of the light is achieved by the cornea, so small changes in the surface of the cornea can have a large effect on how your eye focuses light. The cornea is made of microscopic collagen layers held together like layers of an onion.

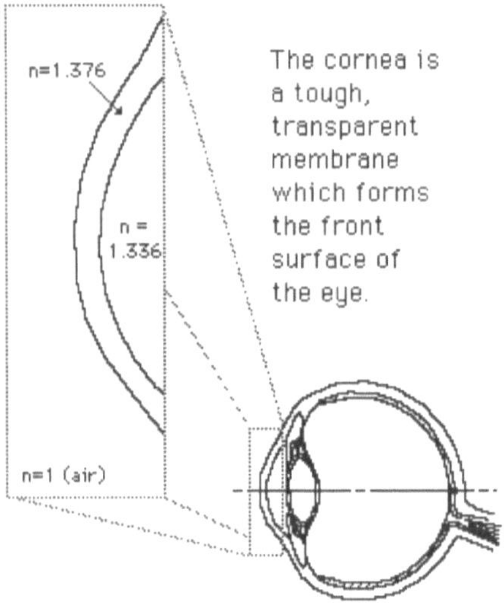

Iris

The iris is the colored part of the eye. The muscles of the iris act to control the size of the pupil.

Pupil

The pupil is the black spot in the center of the iris. The pupil acts to regulate the amount of light that enters the eye. In bright sunlight it becomes smaller letting in less light. In a dark environment the pupil expands to allow more light to reach the retina.

Lens

The lens is a normally clear structure located behind the pupil. It acts to fine tune the focusing. By changing shape, the lens allows us to focus near and far. This ability to focus near (accommodation) gradually worsens with age as the lens gets harder and less supple. Most people notice this in their forties, at which time they begin to need reading glasses or bifocals. As we age, the lens may also become cloudy. This clouding of the lens is called a cataract and may interfere with your vision.

Vitreous

This is the clear gel substance that fills the space between the lens and the retina. If there are opacities in the vitreous, you will see them as "floaters."

Retina

The retina is the thin layer of tissue that lines the inside wall of the eye. It is similar to film in a camera in that it functions to capture and transmit images for interpretation to the brain.

Optic nerve

The optic nerve carries the images from the retina to the brain.

Summary

All of the above are essential parts of the eye that, when normal, function in harmony to insure good vision. When any one of these has some defect or is misshaped, then less than acceptable vision may result.

3
Refractive Error

Vision Problem

THE MOST COMMON VISION PROBLEM is refractive error or the inability of the eye's optics to refract the light properly on the retina. Millions of people worldwide have blurry vision because of some form of refractive error.

There are four types of refractive error: nearsightedness (myopia), farsightedness (hyperopia), astigmatism (oval corneal curvature), and presbyopia (lens becoming less flexible with age).

We can correct refractive error with glasses, contacts, and refractive surgery.

Patients whose vision is still blurry with the best pair of glasses and contacts usually have a vision problem other than refractive error. They may be suffering from cataracts, macular degeneration, or a neurological problem. These problems are typically detected during the eye examination and will require treatment other than refractive surgery.

Fortunately, refractive error is the most common vision impairment and can be easily corrected in most patients with glasses, contacts, or refractive surgery. In fact, most patients' vision can be corrected with Custom LASIK.

Refractive Error

A normal eye should be able to refract (bend) rays of light. In order to see clearly, the optics of the eye, the cornea and the lens, must bend the light in such a way that it focuses on the retina (the back of the eye). If they don't bend the light properly and focus it instead in front of or behind the retina, then we will not see clearly, resulting in a refractive error. When the optics of the eye are too strong, too powerful, they focus the light in front of the retina. We call that nearsightedness or myopia. When the optics are too weak, they focus the light behind the retina. We call that farsightedness or hyperopia. If the cornea is oval instead of round like it's supposed to be, the light focuses in several spots on the retina, instead of one spot. We call that astigmatism. As we get older, usually in our mid-40's, the lens can't accommodate or focus the near objects very well and we need reading glasses. This is called presbyopia.

Glasses and contacts correct sight indirectly. They neutralize the power of the optics but don't correct them permanently. With refractive surgery, we reshape the eye's optics to help them bend the light rays properly, on the retina, to restore clear vision.

Myopia (nearsightedness)

Myopia occurs when the curvature of the cornea is too steep for the length of the eye. As the light rays pass through the steep cornea, they are bent too sharply and come to a point of focus in front of the retina. This creates a blurred image. Patients with myopia are able to see near objects well but have difficulty with their distance vision.

Myopia

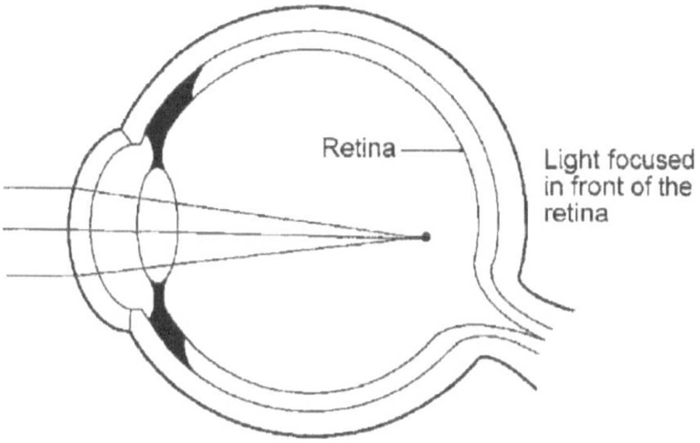

In myopia, nearsightedness, light rays focus in front of the retina, causing distant objects to appear blurry.

With laser vision correction, the cornea is flattened. It can then focus the light more precisely on the retina.

Hyperopia (farsightedness)

Hyperopia occurs when the curvature of the cornea is too flat for the eye. The light rays that enter the eye are not bent sharply enough, causing them to come to a point of focus behind the retina. This produces a blurred image. Farsighted patients see distant objects more clearly than near objects but often have difficulty with both, especially as they get older and the lens can't flex well anymore to counteract the flatness of the cornea.

Some people who are mildly farsighted are able to use the focusing muscle around their lens (accommodation) to bend the light more steeply. This brings the point of focus forward toward the retina and allows them to see more clearly. This ability, however, decreases with age, and reading glasses or bifocals may be needed.

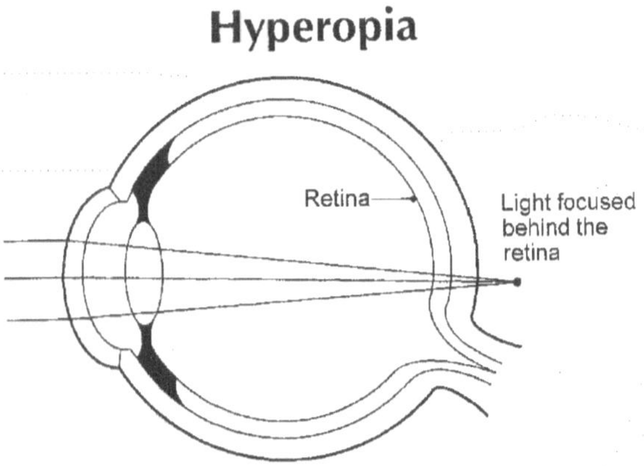

With hyperopia, farsightedness, light rays focus behind the retina. Objects in the distance are seen less blurry than near objects.

Often people who have never worn glasses before find that they start needing them in their forties and fifties. At first they just need them for seeing things up close (presbyopia). However, if the cornea is truly too flat for the length of the eye, a patient will begin to need glasses for distance as well. This phenomenon is called latent hyperopia.

With age, many farsighted individuals not only lose their near vision, they lose their far vision as well and become totally dependent on their glasses or contact lenses at all distances – driving, computer, and reading.

With laser vision correction, the cornea is steepened. It can then focus the light more precisely on the retina.

Astigmatism

Most patients with myopia or hyperopia have some degree of astigmatism. This means that your cornea, rather than being completely spherical like a basketball, is slightly oval and shaped more like a football than a sphere. People with astigmatism experience blurred vision and sometimes distortion or tilting of images due to unequal bending of the rays of light entering their eyes. High degrees of astigmatism will cause blurred vision for both distant and near objects. The image observed on the backside of a spoon is quite distorted and demonstrates a very high degree of astigmatism.

Almost everyone has at least a small amount of astigmatism. For many people, their astigmatism has very little effect on their vision. Unfortunately, the word "astigmatism" is one of those magic words in the English language that almost everyone remembers and is frequently concerned about. The good news is that even the most significant amount of astigmatism can be measurably improved and even completely eliminated with refractive surgery.

Astigmatism

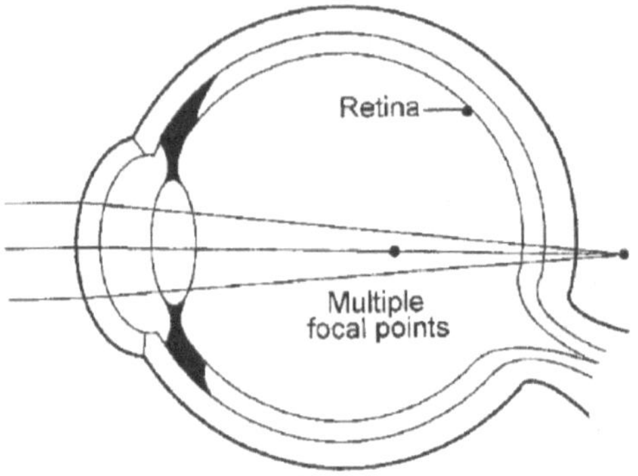

In astigmatism, light entering the eyeball focuses on multiple areas rather than on the retina. Objects both far and near appear blurry.

With laser vision correction, the surgeon makes the cornea more round. It can then focus the light more precisely on the retina.

Measurement of Refractive Errors

You may hear your vision referred to as 20/20 or 20/40 or even 20/400. This is a measurement of your visual acuity using a Snellen chart. The notation 20/40 means you can see at twenty feet what a normal sighted person sees at forty feet (see diagram patient 20/40/60/100ft). These numbers measure your vision but do not quantify your refractive error. There are other variables that affect an interpretation of the chart, such as squinting, guessing at the letters, and room light.

Quantifying your refractive error is done in measurement units called diopters (D). This is the number used to determine your refractive treatment. The more nearsighted or farsighted you are, the worse the vision, and the higher your prescription is in diopters.

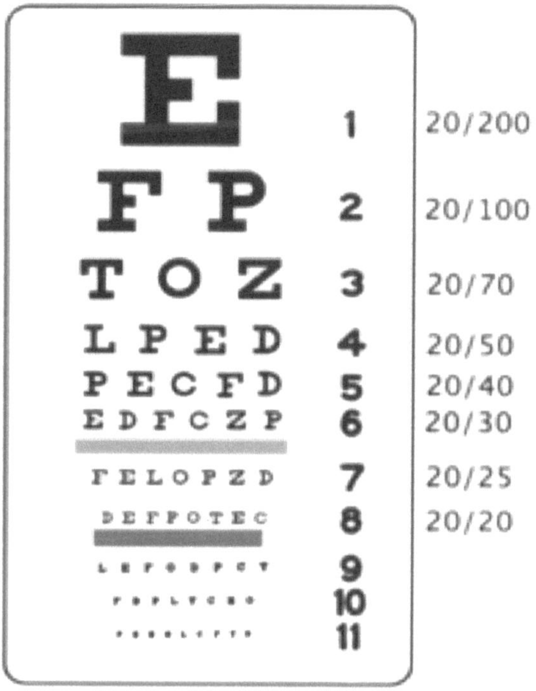

Snellen chart. Illustration not intended for vision testing.

People that are nearsighted (myopic) can see close objects but distant objects are blurred. They require concave lenses in their glasses or contacts to diverge the light rays that are already bent too much by their eye. These refractive errors and corrective lenses are designated by a minus sign in front of the diopter power, for example -3.00 D.

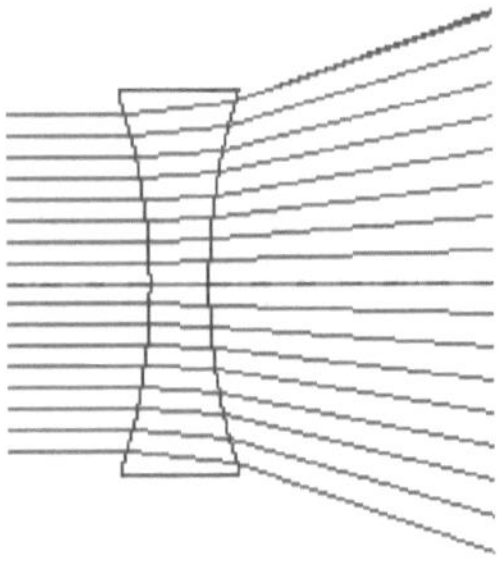

Concave or Negative lenses will diverge (spread out) light rays

People who are farsighted (hyperopic) are lacking refractive or light bending power in their eyes. This lack of refractive power focuses their image behind the retina. They require convex lenses to help converge light. These farsighted refractive errors and corrective lenses are designated by a plus sign in front of the diopter power for example +2.00 D.

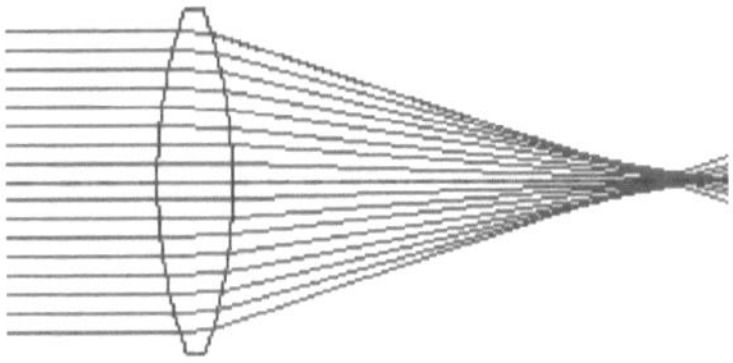

Convex or Positive lenses will converge or focus light and can form an image

You can have mixed lens shapes too, especially if you wear bifocals, trifocals, or progressive glasses.

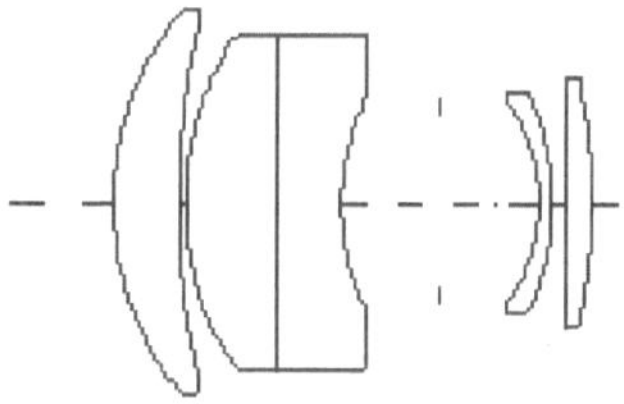

Mixed lens shapes

Your prescription for glasses is typically written in three numbers. For example:
–3.00 –1.25 X 90

The first number (–3.00) identifies your amount of nearsightedness or farsightedness. The sign is an indication of whether you are nearsighted (–) or farsighted (+).

The second number (–1.25) represents your amount of astigmatism.

The third number (90) represents how the astigmatism (or the ovalness of your cornea) is oriented. In this person the astigmatism is at ninety degrees or vertical.

When the eye surgeon corrects your refractive disorder, this prescription will be part of the decision making process in determining the treatment. Your prescription (measured in diopters) forms the basis for the number entered into the computer of the excimer laser. This number determines how much and in what pattern the laser will remove tissue from the cornea. The amount of tissue removed is usually no more than ten percent of the total thickness of the cornea.

Presbyopia

Presbyopia is a normal aging process. It occurs as the protein composition of the lens changes, making it harder and less flexible. As the lens loses its ability to flex, it can no longer bend light rays as sharply, and the ability to focus on near objects is impaired. The onset of presbyopia typically occurs between the age of forty and fifty and continues to worsen through the age of sixty. When this occurs, people who already wear glasses may need bifocals, trifocals, or progressives and those who have never worn glasses may require reading glasses.

Presbyopia is an important concept to understand. The excimer laser has no effect on your eye's focusing muscles or on the lens, so it cannot treat pure presbyopia. Thus, if you only need glasses for reading, refractive surgery usually is not likely to help you unless you choose to have monovision – i.e. one eye mildly nearsighted to help you see objects up close.

Additionally, if you are mildly nearsighted and in your forties, you may notice that while you cannot read clearly with your glasses on, you can read well without them. One advantage of mild myopia is the ability to remove your glasses after presbyopia sets in and still be able to read.

If you are nearsighted and obtain excellent distance vision after undergoing laser vision correction, you will typically become normal sighted. This means that you will lose the ability to read without glasses once presbyopia begins. Like other normal sighted individuals, you will require reading glasses for small print, generally sometime in your forties.

One way to counteract this effect is to keep one eye slightly nearsighted after LASIK. Your mind will automatically use this eye for reading and the fully corrected eye for distance. This is called monovision. You should discuss this possibility with your eye care professional if you are in your late thirties or older.

Why Your Prescription May Look Different at Different Exams

Have you ever wondered why your prescription looks more or less myopic, hyperopic or astigmatic depending on what equipment the doctor uses to check it, if it's a prescription for glasses vs. the numbers on your contact lens box, or if you simply go to a different doctor for a check up.

First of all, your prescription can be written in either "minus" or "plus" astigmatism format, i.e. the astigmatism number has a minus sign. In the above example, it is in the "minus" form. If we were to write it to the "plus" format, i.e. with a "plus" sign in front of the astigmatism number, it would look as follows:

-4.25 + 1.25 x 180

Occasionally, when patients see their prescription written in this form and they are used to seeing it the "minus" form, they become concerned about the first number. They think that this prescription reads much more near-sighted than what they've been at previous examinations. This prescription, however, is identical to the first one. To convert the first prescription into the second prescription, we simply add the first two numbers, preserving their signs, i.e. -3.00 + (-1.25) = -4.25. We then change the sign in front of 1.25 from minus to plus and add 90 to the third number.

The prescription that you get for your eye glasses also looks different from the numbers on your contact lens box. If you are nearsighted, the contact prescription is typically lower, i.e. less "minus" than your eye glass prescription. If you are farsighted, the contact lenses read higher, i.e. more "plus" than your glasses. This discrepancy has to do with how close the corrective lens is to your cornea. The closer it is (i.e. contact lenses), the less “minus” or more “plus” it reads.

When the doctor uses the phoropter during your eye examination - the instrument that looks like Mickey Mouse ears and where you have to look through different lenses and decide which is better “one” or “two” - the prescription that results from that exam is for your eye glasses. This is the prescription that will be used as the basis for your vision correction procedure. However, this prescription will be converted into a different one for contact lenses.

Often, an instrument called autorefractor is used to measure your prescription as well. Typically, it will be used during the initial pre-surgical consultation. You will sit in front of a rectangular box, your chin supported, and will be asked to look at a picture of a distant object, such as a little house projected within the instrument.

Your prescription will print automatically. This prescription will be more similar to your glasses than your contacts. However, it will be only 95% accurate – enough to determine what type of surgical procedure will be best for you, but not accurate enough to determine if your vision has been stable. The doctor will determine the stability of your vision by looking at your old eye glass prescription and comparing it to the current one.

Your prescription may fluctuate from exam to exam. This doesn’t necessarily mean that your prescription is not stable for laser vision correction. Prescription may change from exam to exam because of fluctuations in your tear film, recent contact lens wear, the time of day, how long you worked on your computer prior to the exam, or simply mild physiologic fluctuations in vision. Your surgeon will recommend that you remove contact lenses for a specified period of time prior to your Custom LASIK to help your eyes recover from contact lenses, stabilize the tear film, and your prescription.

Nonsurgical Vision Correction Options

Before considering laser vision correction, you should review the variety of different nonsurgical ways refractive disorders can be corrected. All have benefits and drawbacks.

Glasses

Glasses are time proven and have been in existence for many years. They are affordable (unless you buy multiple pairs of designer frames), easy to maintain, and versatile. They may, however, restrict peripheral vision, be difficult to wear in certain weather conditions, cause images to appear smaller than what they really are, cause a number of visual aberrations (including halos around lights), and have a limited usage life. They may interfere with certain occupations and recreational activities, and some people don't like the cosmetic impact on their appearance. Some people have concerns about safety in an emergency if their glasses are lost or broken.

Contact Lenses

Contact lenses are another common solution for the correction of refractive visual problems. Advantages include more natural vision, no change in cosmetic appearance, more freedom in recreational activities, and better peripheral vision. On the other hand, contacts are high maintenance, may get lost, are less comfortable for patients with dry eyes, may cause visual aberrations (including halos and fluctuating vision), and always carry an increased risk of infection and possible corneal scarring. In higher altitudes many adults become intolerant of contact lenses over time because of dry climate and decreased oxygen in the air.

There are many types of contact lenses available today and the vast majority of people may be fit comfortably, regardless of their level of nearsightedness, farsightedness, or astigmatism.

Orthokeratology

This is a technique that uses a series of rigid contact lenses to flatten your cornea to treat myopia. The effects are not permanent and require continued dependence on part-time retainer lenses. The technique is high maintenance and requires continuous follow-up visits. The long term effects may also lead to permanently warped corneas. The risk of keratitis or infection is also considerably increased over normal contact lens wear.

4
Refractive Surgical Procedures

THE INCREASING NUMBER of refractive procedures developed throughout the world is a testimony to the magnitude of the vision problem. The development of a laser surgical procedure to correct nearsightedness, farsightedness, and astigmatism that is both predictable and relatively safe came into its own in the latter part of the 80's and early 90's and was surely needed. In some parts of the world, the incidence of nearsightedness is close to fifty percent. In the United States alone, as many as seventy-five million people are afflicted with myopia. Additional estimates by the National Institutes of Health report that as many as one adult in four suffers from myopia.

Surgical Procedures

Here are some of the surgical procedures performed today with excellent results:

- Laser in-situ keratomileusis (LASIK)
- Photorefractive keratectomy (PRK)
- Conductive Keratoplasty (CK)
- Laser Thermal Keratoplasty (LTK)
- Intacs™ corneal ring segments
- Implantable Lenses (Phakic IOLs)
- Clear lens extraction (CLE)
- Astigmatic keratotomy (AK)
- Cataract surgery with intraocular lens implantation

The names of these procedures may be hard to pronounce, but the results in correcting poor vision due to refractive errors have been excellent. The high rates of success reported with these procedures—and Custom Lasik in particular—have lead to their widespread acceptance within the ophthalmic community and among patients. Which procedure is right for you will depend on multiple variables:

- Your prescription
- Your corneal thickness and shape
- Your age
- Your eye health

Laser in-situ keratomileusis (LASIK)

LASIK is a surgical procedure intended to reduce a person's dependency on glasses and contacts. It involves two steps: raising the superficial layer of the cornea, called the flap, followed by laser reshaping of the underlying corneal tissue to correct the refractive error.

The formation of the flap is traditionally done with a mechanical bladed device, i.e., microkeratome, or better yet, with a computer guided laser system, i.e., intralase.

Following lifting the flap, a computer controlled excimer laser then delivers overlapping pulses of cool ultraviolet light to underlying corneal tissue, removing or "evaporating" microscopic layers. Once the reshaping is done, then the flap is folded back on the eye where it self-seals within seconds. The entire procedure takes approximately five minutes.

Photorefractive Keratotomy (PRK)

PRK was the first FDA approved laser refractive procedure. During this procedure, the surgeon uses an excimer laser to reshape the outer surface of the cornea to treat your optical prescription. Unlike LASIK, no flap is created. The reshaping laser is applied directly to the surface of the cornea. Often, the wavefront map of your vision is used to guide the laser treatment, just as in the second step of LASIK. The results are identical to LASIK, but vision recovers slower. Sometimes it is referred to as the no flap LASIK.

Generally, this technique is reserved for patients who have thin corneas, are apprehensive about LASIK, or have a history of other refractive procedures. Your eye surgeon can advise you accordingly.

Conductive Keratoplasty (CK)

CK is a procedure approved by the FDA for the temporary reduction of hyperopia or presbyopia in patients over 40 years of age. CK uses radio frequency energy to reshape the cornea and make it more curved or more nearsighted. It is safe and effective and takes only a few minutes. Other alternatives to CK include glasses, contact lenses, PRK, LASIK or LTK. The magnitude of correction may diminish over time.

Laser Thermal Keratoplasty (LTK)

LTK is a laser procedure that is referred to as no touch. This procedure corrects mild degrees of farsightedness. Heat is applied to the periphery of the cornea to shrink the peripheral collagen, indirectly steepening the cornea centrally. The procedure is non-invasive but has a tendency to regress. Its outcomes may also be less accurate than LASIK or PRK to treat the farsightedness. It is performed in select cases.

Intacs

Intacs are special inserts that are placed into the periphery of the corneas to induce flattening. The procedure is reversible by removing the inserts. This is a technique that is not commonly used to treat myopia. It is used in treating certain cases of corneal thinning, such as keratoconus. With Intacs, we can help these patients see better and often avoid a corneal transplant.

Implantable Contact Lenses (Phakic IOLs)

Unlike wearing a regular contact lens on the outside of the cornea, with the implantable contact lens, an ultra thin lens, designed to correct nearsightedness or farsightedness, is permanently placed behind the cornea. This procedure is not for everyone. It is indicated for patients with extreme nearsightedness and farsightedness. For select patients, it works exceptionally well. Your surgeon will direct you accordingly.

Astigmatic Keratotomy (AK)

With Astigmatic Keratotomy, the surgeon places one or two incisions at the periphery of the cornea to relax it into a more spherical shape. AK is typically performed in conjunction with another eye surgery, such as cataract surgery. It may also be performed after a corneal transplant. For most patients with astigmatism, the condition can be easily treated with Custom LASIK.

Cataract Surgery with Intraocular Lens Implantation

As part of the aging process, the crystalline lens gets cloudy, thus interfering with distance or near vision. The surgeon can replace the cloudy lens with a clear plastic lens which is also designed to correct nearsightedness or farsightedness. Significant advances in cataract surgery have also brought us lenses that can help elderly patients see well for far and near, thus reducing dependence on both distance and reading glasses. Traditionally the intraocular lens is monofocal or fixed-focus; however, recently there have been some new multifocal or accommodating lenses that allow the patient to see clearly distance and close vision. The procedure is performed in an outpatient surgery center under a local, topical anesthetic with a no-stitch microincision. A special A-scan measurement is required to select the desired intraocular lens power. With an excellent, experienced surgeon, the recovery is quick, painless, and rewarding.

Often, the vision can be "fine tuned" after cataract surgery with Custom LASIK. As long as the eyes are healthy, there is no upper age limit.

Clear Lens Extraction (CLE)

Clear lens extraction is recommended for patients who do not qualify for LASIK due to severe farsightedness, nearsightedness, thin corneas, or cataract formation. With CLE, the patient's natural crystalline lens is removed and replaced with a special intraocular lens similar to cararact surgery.

Former Refractive Surgery Procedures

Automated Lamellar Keratoplasty (ALK)

ALK is a surgical procedure developed in the mid-eighties to correct vision. The outer layer of the cornea is raised by a microkeratome creating a flap, followed by another pass over the cornea to reshape it. The LASIK concept was derived from ALK and has gained grounds for better precision and accuracy.

Radial Keratotomy

RK was a popular procedure in the 70s. Established by Professor Fydorov in Moscow, it used to be the only procedure available to correct nearsightedness and astigmatism. With this procedure, multiple radial incisions were placed onto the anterior surface of the cornea to flatten it. Regression and over correction with issues of weakening of the cornea were noted. In the mid 90s, it was replaced by the more accurate laser vision correction.

Patients who still need to wear glasses after having had RK in the past, can have their vision corrected with Custom LASIK.

While there are many types of refractive surgery, we are focusing primarily on Custom LASIK. This procedure has proved to be highly effective and safe for most ranges of nearsightedness, farsightedness, and astigmatism and is readily accepted by both patients and doctors today.

5
LASIK and the Latest Advancements

LASIK IS A TWO-STEP PROCESS that has been performed on millions of patients and it has proven to be safe and effective. In the last several years, however, two revolutionary advances have taken place in LASIK surgery. These two advances have added a new level of safety and precision to the procedure, compelling more patients than ever and even more eye doctors than ever to undergo LASIK vision correction.

The first advance is the Intralase femtosecond laser which is now slowly replacing the traditional, hand held mechanical device used to lift the superficial layer of the cornea called the flap. This step is necessary to expose the inner layers of the cornea where the reshaping laser, called the excimer laser, will be applied to reshape the cornea, correcting nearsightedness, farsightedness, and astigmatism.

The second advance in LASIK eye surgery is the Wavefront Scan. With this mapping system, we can now record the unique patterns in each person's vision system, transfer these maps to the excimer laser, and then use these maps to guide the laser in correcting each person's unique vision imperfections.

Intralase femtosecond laser and Wavefront Scan driven excimer laser, form the foundation of Custom LASIK. Both components are essential for a truly customized LASIK.

Step One: Flap Formation

In traditional LASIK, the flap is created with a mechanical device called a microkeratome which utilizes a metal blade. With a microkeratome, the superficial cornea is cut, forming a microthin layer that is hinged superiorly or nasally. Although microkeratomes are safe and accurate, they rarely lead to problems that can affect vision. Even in the hands of experienced surgeons, microkeratome can rarely result in incomplete flaps, button hole flaps, thickness variations, and even corneal abrasions. Often in such situations the LASIK procedure is postponed and completed at a later time.

All that changed with the advent of the Intralase femtosecond laser. With the Intralase femtosecond laser, the surgeon focuses the laser beam at the preset depth in the cornea. Each laser pulse creates a microscopic air bubble. Thousands of these tiny air bubbles are precisely delivered to lift the superficial corneal layer of the exact diameter, thickness, and placement needed to accommodate each individual's unique eye anatomy.

Patients with thinner corneas, flatter corneas, more curved corneas, and patients with smaller eyes can now have the procedure done with more safety and precision.

The Intralase doesn't slide across the cornea like the mechanical microkeratome. Therefore, the chance of getting a corneal abrasion during the procedure is reduced.

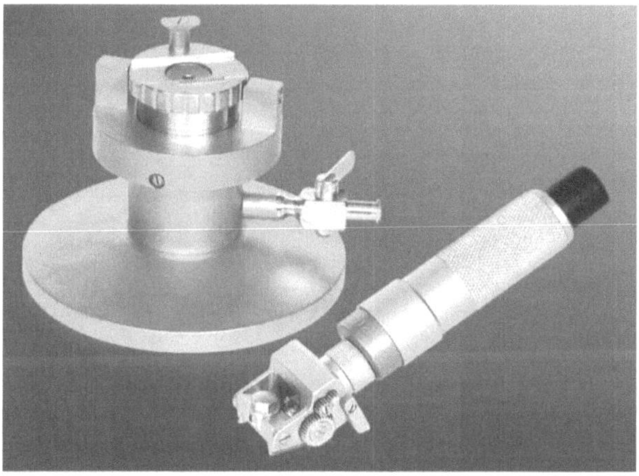

Microkeratome

Studies have demonstrated increased safety and accuracy with the Intralase femtosecond laser compared with the mechanical microkeratome.

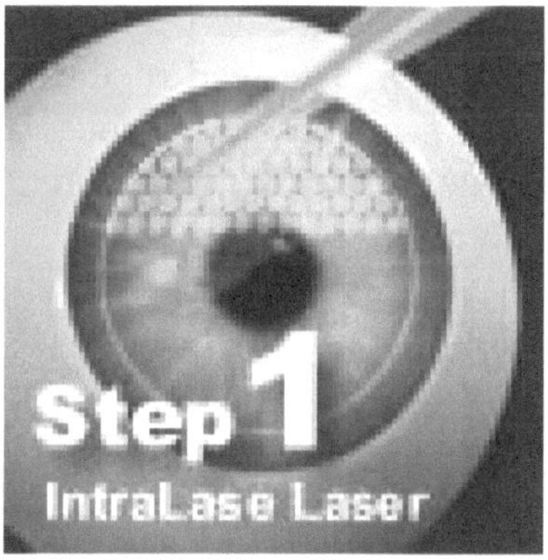

In Step One, a micro-thin flap is created. Thousands of laser pulse bubbles are connected together in a raster pattern to separate the flap from the cornea. In step two, the excimer laser is applied to remove very tiny amounts of tissue to reshape the cornea.

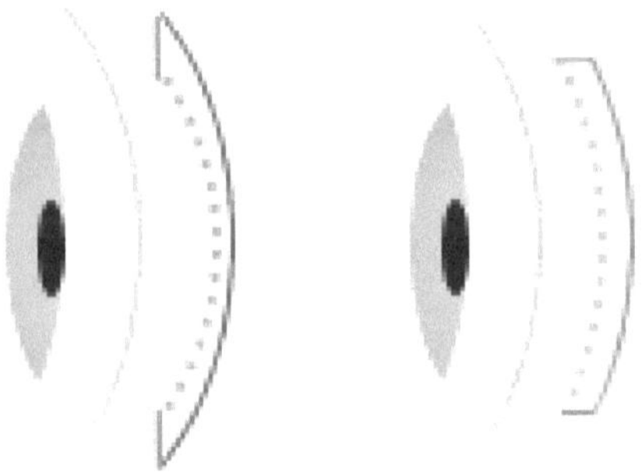

Intralase femtosecond laser advantages:

- Uniform flap thickness
- Uniform flap bed
- Round flap with beveled edge for precise repositioning, alignment, and seating of the flap

In certain instances, the surgeon may prefer to use the mechanical microkeratome instead of the Intralase. Patients who have significant scars on their corneas and patients with previous radial keratotomy (RK) are better candidates for the mechanical microkeratome.

Step Two: Custom Reshaping

Just prior to the second step, the surface layer (the flap) is lifted to expose the inner corneal layers. The surgeon then uses the excimer laser to reshape the inner cornea. The excimer laser beam is guided by the Wavefront map of your vision. This map is typically performed on the day of your procedure, but could also be done at the preoperative exam or both. The map is electronically transferred to the excimer laser just prior to the procedure. It then guides the laser beam during the procedure to correct your vision, i.e., nearsightedness, farsightedness, and astigmatism, as well as smaller imperfections that often affect your night vision. In reshaping your cornea, the excimer laser will vaporize tiny amounts of the corneal tissue. The exact pattern of how the cornea is reshaped will depend on the Wavefront map. In a nearsighted patient, the cornea will be flattened. In a farsighted patient, the cornea will be steepened. And in a patient with astigmatism, the cornea will be made rounder. As a result, the optics of the vision system will be improved so that the images can focus more perfectly on the retina.

Studies have shown that Wavefront-guided corneal reshaping often improves night vision, reduces the incidence of glare and halos at night, and improves contrast sensitivity.

The following diagrams illustrate how the flap is moved aside and computer assisted surgery is performed by a beam of laser light guided by the Wavefront map and controlled by the eye surgeon.

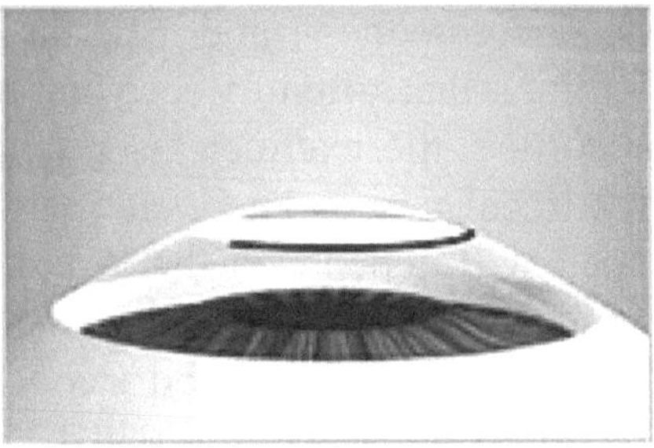

On the surface of the eye (cornea), a thin flap is created.

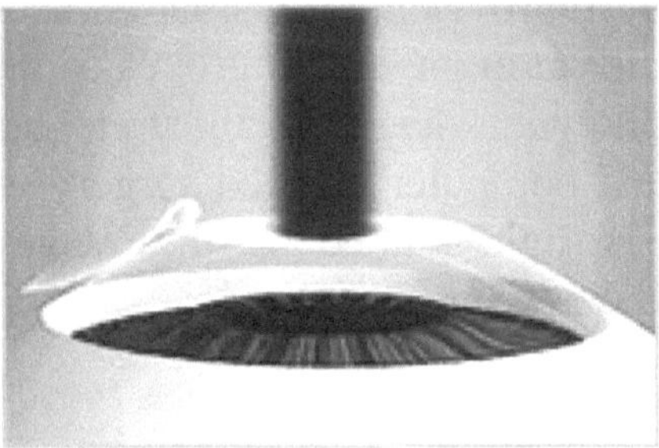

Computer assisted, the eye surgeon releases laser energy to reshape the cornea.

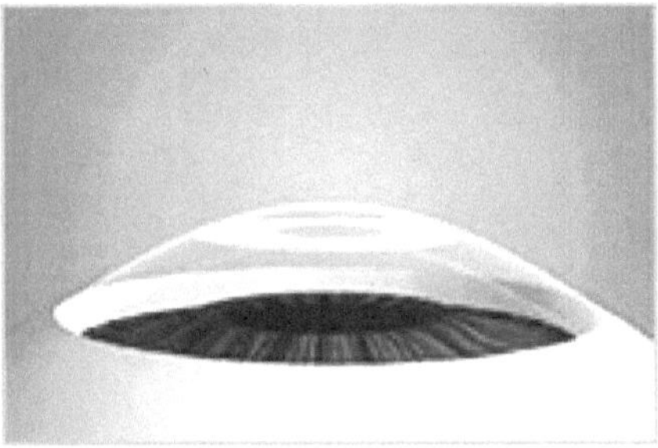

Once reshaped, the flap is replaced and the body seals it shut for rapid recovery of much improved vision

With Custom LASIK, we have refined the art of better vision for our patients. With the new generation of lasers, we can offer unprecedented safety and accuracy and give the world an astounding advance in medicine that until recent years was hardly imagined.

6
Wavefront

WAVEFRONT MAPPING OF YOUR VISION is an essential component of the Custom LASIK procedure. It will first direct the surgeon in deciding if you will benefit from the wavefront-guided laser vision correction. It then guides the laser in reshaping your vision according to the unique patterns in your vision map.

Wavefront technology was originally developed to be in high powered telescopes to reduce distortions when viewing distant objects in space. It was only a matter of time before scientists applied the precision of wavefront technology to reduce distortions in human vision. Prior to Wavefront technology, doctors could only measure the larger imperfections in a patient's vision — nearsightedness, farsightedness, and astigmatism. Therefore, we could help patients see as good as they did with glasses or contacts. Today, we can measure and correct the unique imperfections in vision and provide better vision than glasses or contacts.

How Does Wavefront Mapping Work?

Prior to your Custom LASIK procedure, the Wavefront Mapping of your vision will be performed. You will be seated in front of a high tech device, called a Wavefront Aberrometer, and asked to look at the red target light in front of you.

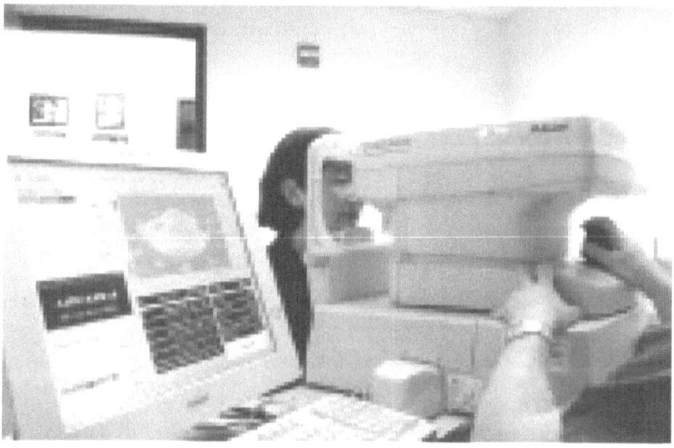

Alcon Advanced Wavefront Mapping with the Wavefront Aberrometer

A harmless infrared laser beam will be sent through the cornea and the lens to the retina. This beam of laser light will then be reflected back through the eye's optical structures. The image of the reflected beam will be captured by a sensor. The sensor inputs the data into the computer that applies a mathematical formula to create a 3-D map of your vision based on the image of the reflected beam. This 3-D map is your Wavefront map.

The map will contain the unique pattern of irregularities in your eye's optical structures — large irregularities such as nearsightedness, farsightedness, and astigmatism, as well as small irregularities that can diminish the quality of your vision if they are present in significant amounts. These irregularities or imperfections are called aberrations. Large imperfections are called lower order aberrations and small imperfections are called higher order aberrations.

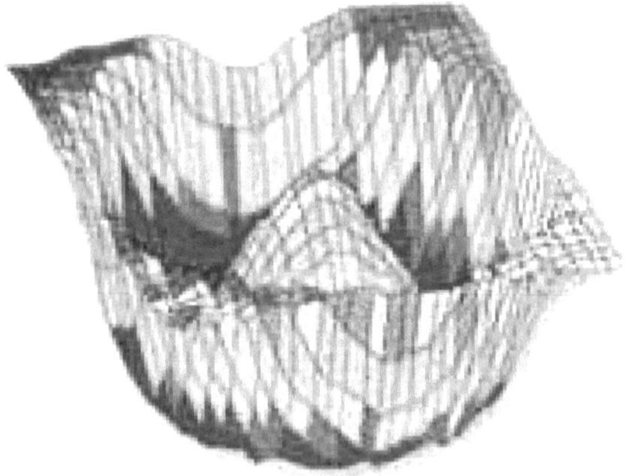

The scan shown here is the 3-D map of the reflected wavefront. This is a fingerprint of your vision, or a map. This information is then transferred to the excimer laser and is used as a guide to reshape the cornea during your Custom LASIK treatment

How Is Wavefront-guided Custom LASIK done?

First, we analyze your wavefront map and compare the results to all the other vision tests that were performed during your preprocedural examination. An important test during your examination is your Refraction, i.e., when we place you in front of the phoropter ("Mickey Mouse glasses") and ask you which is better, "one" or "two"? This test measures how your brain interprets the prescription in your eyes' optics.

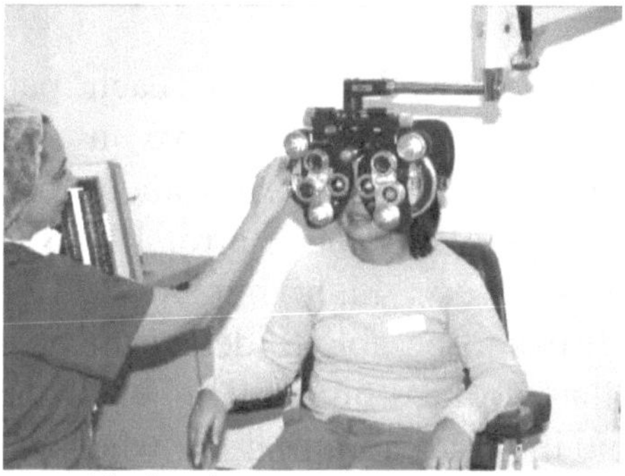

Refraction with the phoropter is an important step in the Custom LASIK process

In most patients, however, the wavefront map and refraction prescriptions are similar and wavefront-guided LASIK is an excellent option if you are one of them.

Once the mapping is completed, the aberrometer software creates a custom tailored treatment map and the information is delivered to the excimer system to reshape the cornea. Most excimer lasers have the ability for active tracking and iris registration to ensure centered treatment. The excimer laser is a cool ultraviolet laser that vaporizes tiny corneal particles to reshape the cornea.

The reshaping pattern will be based on the 3-D wavefront pattern to correct the imperfections in your vision that will include both your lower order aberrations and your higher order aberrations.

Four T's to Successful Custom LASIK

We have developed a system called the "4 T's to Successful Custom LASIK": Technology, Technique, Tear Film, and Team. All four components must be in place with precision accuracy to achieve superb results.

Technology

The aberrometer needs to capture each patient's unique wavefront accurately. Patients have a wide range of prescriptions and therefore the aberrometer has to be able to detect a wide range of refractive errors that range from very high myopia to very high hyperopia, and significant astigmatism. It has to be able to detect the aberrations when the pupil dilates over 5mm. Higher order aberrations primarily come into play in dim light, when the pupil dilates. The aberrometer needs to detect and measure these peripheral aberrations in order for them to be treated.

Studies show that if the aberrations are not measured, they are not treated. The aberrometer also needs to detect many different types of higher order aberrations. While the spherical aberration and coma are the most significant contributors to glare at night, many other types of higher order aberrations contribute as well. Therefore, the aberrometer needs to detect as many as possible so that they can be treated to maximize the quality of vision.

And lastly, the lens in the eye needs to be neutralized for accurate wavefront measurements. Under normal circumstances the lens of the eye tends to overreact and accommodate. To off-set such an induced reaction, your doctor may need to dilate the pupil to relax the lens in order to obtain precise measurements. Treating an accommodating eye may result in blurred vision due to overcorrection or undercorrection. Therefore, it is essential to acquire wavescan measurements when the patient is in a nonaccommodative state.

The Wavefront map is performed with the patient sitting upright in front of the aberrometer. The corneal reshaping is performed with the patient lying down under the excimer laser. In many patients, the eyes rotate when they change body position from upright to lying down. This eye rotation is called cyclotorsion. The wavefront map, with its specific pattern of imperfections, has to match the eye surface for accurate treatment, much like Pringles potato chips have to fit perfectly together or otherwise crumble. Even a ten degree mismatch between the map of the eye and the position of the eye can lead to significant inaccuracies in treating vision imperfections. In fact, the imperfections may increase rather than decrease.

Therefore, an accurate wavefront system has to have provisions to match the map of the eye in a sitting and supine position to avoid cyclotorsion.

The final critical component of the technology essential for accurate wavefront-guided treatment is the excimer laser itself. It has to have an ultra-fast tracker, a tiny beam that treats a wide area of aberrations. In a study published in *Journal of Refractive Surgery*, researchers found that to accurately follow and track the eye during treatment, the tracker has to sample the position of the eye at least 1000 times per second. Less than that and the eye will not be tracked accurately. The scientists also found that as the beam diameter gets smaller, more imperfections can be treated, much like an artist can paint fine detail better with a fine tip brush. Ideal beam diameter is less than one mm.

The size of the treatment zone also matters. As the pupil dilates widely at night, a large treatment zone ensures that most of the light enters through the corrected cornea, reducing risk of glare at night. If the treatment zone is small, such as 6 mm, and the pupil dilates to 8 mm, some light will enter through the 2mm ring of uncorrected cornea and the patient will experience more glare at night.

Technique

A profound, sterile technique is very essential for success of the surgery. Your doctor may elect to start you on antibiotic drops prior to the procedure.

Formation of a good, healthy flap is safer done with an intralase versus a blade guided system; at the end of the procedure, one should make sure that the flap is folded back, aligned and sealed to avoid slippage.

Technology alone is not enough to achieve successful Custom LASIK. Meticulous technique is essential to accurately acquire, match, and treat vision aberrations. All the data points have to be mapped. Excellent correlation between wavefront refraction and phoropter refraction needs to be achieved. Meticulous alignment between the wavefront map and the eye surface needs to be maintained during treatment.

Tear Film

Tear film is part of the eye's optics. Therefore, stable tear film is required for the accurate wavefront map. It is recommended that patients remove their contact lenses prior to their Custom LASIK procedure for the duration of time prescribed by their eye doctor. Some patients may need to use lubricating drops two to four times a day while out of contacts. Some patients may require other interventions to stabilize their tear film prior to the procedure. In some patients, the tear film will never stabilize enough for accurate wavefront mapping and the best procedure for them will be refraction-based correction rather than wavefront-based correction. In any case, your tear film needs to be evaluated during the initial consultation so that appropriate recommendations can be made.

Team

High caliber technical personnel, in addition to the experienced surgeon, is required to integrate complex technology with these meticulous techniques. Extensive training, background in eye care, and even background in computer technology are often necessary.

How to Analyze Published Data and FDA Studies

An essential concern of patients, besides having an expert surgeon with the skill needed to accurately perform Custom LASIK, is the technology track record.

Different technology platforms are often compared in terms of percent of patients who see 20/40 or 20/20 or better after the procedure. For example, you may read that with laser X 95% of patients saw 20/20 or better six months after the procedure while with laser Y 79% of patients saw 20/20 or better. Does this mean that laser X is better than laser Y? Not at all! In order to compare the two lasers, you have to make sure that you are comparing apples to apples, not apples to oranges.

First, you have to make sure that the lasers were used to treat patients with similar amounts of refractive error. Clearly, patients with -2 D myopia are more likely to achieve 20/20 after procedure than patients with -10 D myopia. If patients treated with laser X had lower prescriptions than patients treated with laser Y, then they would be more likely to achieve 20/20. Compare mean preoperative refractive error, standard deviation, and the range of refraction treated.

Additionally, compare the number of patients at the follow-up time point when the results are compared. If only half the original patient sample treated with laser X showed up for a follow-up exam six months after the procedure compared to laser Y, then the data may be artificially skewed in the laser X sample.

Also, analyze the reason why more patients achieved 20/20 with laser X. It could simply be that there was no refractive error left postoperatively with laser X, whereas a little bit of nearsightedness, for example -0.50D was left over with laser Y. This means that the surgeon using laser Y can simply add extra 0.50 D to each treatment and the results will be the same as with laser X. This is called a simple "nomogram adjustment" and can be easily incorporated into the programmed treatment plan, making the results of laser X and laser Y the same.

In fact, if you take into account the statistical differences and nomogram adjustments and then compare the 20/20 outcomes of all the wavefront laser platforms currently approved by the FDA, you will realize that the results are, in fact, similar. They seem better in some platforms, mainly because fewer patients came in for follow-up exams.

The real test of the wavefront-guided Custom LASIK treatment is how well higher order aberrations are recorded. Diagnosing the higher order aberrations and improving the quality of vision is the real purpose of wavefront-guided Custom LASIK. In fact, with these wavefront laser systems, the chance of you having fewer imperfections in your vision than you had with glasses or contact lenses is five times better with the wavefront-guided Custom LASIK than with the conventional procedure. Make sure to ask your surgeon if he or she uses the system that has been shown to reduce higher order aberrations in clinical trials.

The currently FDA approved "wavefront guided" lasers are:

- Visx
- Bausch and Lomb
- Ladar Vision

Although the surgeon cannot promise 20/20 vision without correction, historically ninety-five percent of typical myopic patients achieve vision within two or three lines of 20/20 vision without correction. In fact, the vast majority of patients can drive without glasses the day after their Custom LASIK surgery. With Custom LASIK, great day and night vision is now within your reach.

7

Selecting the Right LASIK Surgeon

THE KEYS TO SUCCESSFUL, safe surgery in any field of medicine are an informed patient with realistic expectations and a skilled, experienced surgeon. Take the time to research the surgeon and the laser team that you are considering for correcting your vision. *Ask questions!* The following guidelines will help you in your quest.

Begin with People You Know

A word-of-mouth network often provides a good initial source of information. Ask your eye doctor. Your eye doctor is critical in your decision making process. First of all, he or she is familiar with your prescription and your vision needs. Also, the doctor is able to evaluate the surgeon's work first hand with at least several patients and compare the work by different surgeons. Your eye doctor should have your best interests in mind. He or she will only recommend what's best for you. Also, ask family, friends, and associates if they could recommend a surgeon based on personal experience.

It is imperative that you have the conviction that your LASIK surgeon will treat you with your best interest at heart. A high quality eye surgeon who has successfully treated other eye doctors, friends and family is usually a good bet.

Consult Physician Directories

Physician search directories available on the Internet may be helpful. Keep in mind, however, that these directories are not exhaustive listings of all the refractive surgeons in your area, only those who have chosen to participate in them. Some directories are new and have a limited number of listings; other directories charge a fee for listing the surgeon's name.

Keep in mind, too, that the majority of these sites and their referrals do not check a surgeon's credentials. So make sure you thoroughly research a surgeon's credentials before making the final decision.

Contact Ophthalmic Boards and Medical Associations

Ophthalmic boards and medical associations offer useful information about board certification, licensing, and other pertinent criteria. Among the better known entities are the American Academy of Ophthalmology, the American Society of Cataract and Refractive Surgery, and the International Society of Refractive Surgery.

You should contact your local or national ophthalmic associations for their lists of member surgeons. Be sure to contact more than one professional organization, as not all ophthalmologists are members of each one. Even if you have heard of good surgeons from a friend, relative, or acquaintance, take the time to check their professional credentials.

What to Look for

Board Certification

Always look for a board certified physician. This is the medical profession's generally accepted form of accreditation. This information can be obtained from the American Academy of Ophthalmology or the American Medical Association (AMA). The surgeon must be fellowship trained in corneal diseases and refractive surgery.

Experience with the Procedure

You would like a surgeon who has been doing refractive surgery for at least three years. Experience in dealing with different patients' refractive needs and surgical results over time are most valuable and cannot be overstated. The more experience a surgeon has the better. Refractive surgery is both an art and a science, including assessing different patients' needs before surgery, performing the surgery with great attention to detail, following the healing process, and intervening (if necessary) postoperatively. Refractive techniques and technology change over time. This experience imparts to the surgeon a comprehensive understanding of the surgical process and enables him or her to satisfy each patient's needs.

Numerous studies have shown that surgeons experience a learning curve with the LASIK procedure. It has been shown that surgeons who have performed over 1000 procedures have a lower complication rate than those who have performed fewer. Generally, it could take approximately 200 LASIK procedures before your surgeon is able to develop a fine adjustment of this final treatment plan. It is based on a series of measurements performed at the time of the preoperative exam, as well as on the surgeon's technique and the laser used. A well developed adjustment allows the surgeon to more accurately program the laser for each patient, decreasing the probability that an enhancement procedure will be necessary. You need to be aware, however, that even in the best hands, enhancement procedures are necessary five percent of the time. Different people can have a small variance in response to the laser, in particular those with higher prescriptions are more likely to need an enhancement.

In the process of performing these procedures, the surgeon should make every effort to meet or exceed benchmark standards in order to achieve good outcomes. By constantly analyzing surgical outcomes, the better surgeons find that the consistency of their results improves, even beyond the initial 1,000 procedures.

Find out how much experience the surgeon has with your procedure. Ask if they have a nomogram. Ask to see it. Ask how frequently they update it.

Do not be deceived by a laser center that has done several thousand procedures. It is the surgeon that makes a difference.

Tracking Results

As a potential patient, you should ask your doctor how he or she tracks LASIK procedure outcomes. The doctor's response can tell you a great deal. If the surgeon has done extensive work developing excimer laser technology, presents his or her data at well respected conferences to other surgeons, or publishes, you can be confident that he or she is tracking their results.

Because there is no mandatory central reporting database for tracking results, the important thing is to determine if the surgeon is tracking and not worry too much about any one specific number. The fact that the surgeon is tracking LASIK outcomes shows his or her concern for achieving the best possible results. Your goal is to find someone for whom achieving excellence is a paramount concern.

Success and Complication Rates

Next, ask the surgeons how long they have been performing refractive surgery and Custom LASIK and about their success and complication rates. Your doctor should discuss the potential success rate for your individual surgery, as well as any potential complications. Surgical success means more than knowing how to avoid complications; it means knowing how to handle difficult situations before they arise. Identifying problems early and dealing with them in a timely manner is the hallmark of excellent surgeons. All surgeons have complications, but that does not mean that anything was done wrong. What is important is that the surgeon has a low complication rate and that the ultimate visual outcomes are good.

It is also important to know about their experience with refractive errors similar to your own. The surgeons should have adequate experience with people of the same age, gender, and race as you because the surgical techniques needed to correct refractive errors in these groups may differ slightly from the norm.

Computerized Corneal Topography

Computerized corneal topography is a valuable tool in kerato-refractive surgery. With this technology, the surgeon measures the surface contour of the cornea, which is responsible for approximately seventy five percent of the refractive power of your eye. Color digital pictures generated from these measurements demonstrate a patient's degree of corneal curvature, astigmatism, or any irregularities measured at approximately 7,000 points across the cornea. These maps allow the surgeon to see all the details of a patient's astigmatism and whether the astigmatism is symmetric, asymmetric, or irregular in nature. They also allow the doctor to observe some incipient (just beginning to appear) corneal diseases that may not otherwise be clinically detectable, such as early keratoconus.

These maps define corneal surface contour in great detail. They are especially valuable for use in patients with difficult astigmatism. Computerized corneal topography is also helpful with the enhancement surgery when the surgeon assesses the features of the patient's prior treatment. Utilizing the information from these maps, the surgeon can customize his or her treatment to each individual patient.

More advanced topographic systems are the orbscan and the pentacam. Such technologies provide your surgeon an extensive amount of information pertaining to the anterior surface of the cornea, the back surface of the cornea, steeping of the cornea and the thickness of the cornea (pachymetry). The orbscan and pentacam systems have changed the world of refractive surgery because they can precisely detect abnormalities that the physician was unable to detect with the standard topography system.

Enhancement Policy

An enhancement surgery is any follow-up laser treatment after the first surgery to further improve a patient's vision. How liberal or stringent is the surgeon's policy on enhancement surgery? Some of the offices may not allow enhancement procedures to further improve uncorrected vision (vision measured without contact lenses or glasses) unless a patient sees 20/50 or worse.

For instance, after the first procedure your uncorrected vision is 20/40 and your desire for an enhancement to further improve your vision may not be allowed. Even though most people can pass their drivers test with 20/40 vision, some patients may not be happy with this level of vision for their distance acuity.

Prior to making a decision to have refractive surgery, it is important to understand the center's policy for allowing you to have enhancement surgery. Do they allow enhancements only if your uncorrected vision is 20/50 or worse? Also, what if your vision is 20/40, 20/30, or 20/25 after the first surgery and you want it improved? Will they allow an enhancement under your global fee since they corrected you to 20/40 or better? Will you be charged for an enhancement? What exactly is their policy? Always feel free to ask.

Beware of "Lifetime Guarantee"

With "Lifetime Guarantee", you may be promised enhancements free of charge "for life." Often, many exclusions apply. For example, enhancements for farsightedness (hyperopia) may be excluded. You may need to have yearly exams after your procedure to qualify for free enhancements. And while you should have your eye health checked yearly, sometimes you may be traveling or living outside the US and not be able to come back in a year for a check up. What if you come in a year and a half later? Will "Lifetime Guarantee" still apply? What if you have glare at night and need a wavefront-guided enhancement, or custom upgrade? "Lifetime Guarantee" often excludes these and you may have to pay an additional fee for this type of enhancement.

Excimer Laser Capability

The computer software that operates the excimer laser varies from manufacturer to manufacturer. And while all excimer lasers have the software necessary to perform simple treatments, not all have the advanced wavefront capabilities. In selecting a surgeon and a laser center, make certain that the doctor's laser has the capability of correcting your vision using your wavefront map. You may hear "wavefront optimized" or "custom". These terms don't necessarily mean that the laser platform is capable of wavefront-guided treatments. Ask the doctor specifically about wavefront-guided treatment.

Awareness of New Developments

Most doctors keep up with the latest developments by reading or attending conferences. Some doctors take this a step further and immerse themselves in a life style of innovation by lecturing at major conferences, teaching surgical technique to other doctors, participating in clinical trials for new technology, and consulting for ophthalmology companies.

Ask the doctors you talk to if they know what is being achieved, both nationally and internationally, in their field. Or contact one of the major ophthalmologic societies directly with the same question.

Personal Compatibility

Remember, personal chemistry is extremely important. Choose a doctor with whom you feel comfortable; someone who is easy to talk to, friendly, and professional; someone who listens closely to what you want and cares about what you need. Make sure he or she is willing to take the time necessary for your understanding of the procedure. A good doctor-patient relationship is important in helping devise a treatment plan that best suits your needs.

The art of medicine entails blending the science of medicine with the needs and expectations of the individual patient. Many excellent LASIK surgeons and LASIK centers offer consultations that give you an opportunity to assess the quality and excellence levels of the person to whom you are entrusting your eyes.

Competent, Compassionate Staff

Verify that the laser center is staffed with highly trained, competent professionals. Determine for yourself whether the LASIK surgeon has the competent team to insure an excellent outcome for you. Here are some questions that may help you find the right team:

- Does the surgeon work with other eye care professionals to assist in patient examinations?
- Does the surgeon have technical support for lasers and the advanced technology?
- Have any of them had refractive surgery with the surgeon?
- Does your prospective surgeon have his own laser onsite, or does he share with a group of other surgeons at another location?
- Does he have a laser brought into his office or other center on surgery days?
- Does it appear overall that the surgeon has made a significant commitment to excimer laser and LASIK surgery?
- Does the surgeon have a doctor(s) working with him that specializes or spends most of their time working with preoperative and postoperative LASIK patients?
- Do they understand your needs?

- What is their experience and role in the delivery of your care?
- Have they had LASIK surgery?
- Who will be doing the surgery?

Care Provider and Style of Care
Determine who will be performing your pre-operative and post-operative care. Many patients choose to see their family optometrist or ophthalmologist for their preoperative and/or post-operative care. Such an arrangement is known as co-management. It can enhance the overall level of your care. The co-managing doctor is often familiar with your previous eye history, your prescriptions, your lifestyle, and the best correction that works for you. This information can help your surgeon tremendously in optimizing your surgical result.

Find a Qualified Surgeon

Find an experienced LASIK surgeon who will make the commitment to you to take full responsibility to give you the best possible result from LASIK and who will be actively involved in every aspect of your LASIK procedure.

Be sure you know who is actually doing the procedure. Ask who will be doing your follow-up. Ask about their qualifications. Find out how many procedures he or she has done. While higher volume does not necessarily imply a better surgeon, you will want someone who has done at least several thousand surgeries. Ask what his or her success rate is for 20/20 vision or better. What is his or her rate of loss of best corrected vision?

Remember, when evaluating the criteria you feel that a LASIK surgeon should meet, take time to listen to your feelings. This is one sure way to feel comfortable with the surgeon you finally select. At any point in the decision making process, should you have doubts about the surgeon or his or her medical assessment, go elsewhere and obtain a second opinion.

Ask How Many LASIK Procedures the Surgeon Has Performed

It is important to be specific with regard to LASIK since many surgeons have performed other laser procedures that require different skills than those required for LASIK. Just because the surgeon has done thousands of retinal or glaucoma procedures does not mean that he or she has done many LASIK procedures.

Does the Surgeon Maintain a Database of a number of LASIK Procedures?

This database will allow the surgeon to provide you with statistics regarding his or her results. Specifically, the surgeon will be able to provide you with a reasonable prediction of what your result will be (based on your preoperative refraction) and the likelihood of needing an enhancement procedure to fine tune your result.

Choose the Right Surgeon and Pay What It Costs

Discount surgery is as good as a discount parachute. Many advertisements push low cost surgery. This is an important warning signal to proceed with caution. Go for the best qualified surgeon and the treatment team.

Beware of the Hard Sell

Be wary of promises or guarantees seen in advertisements, such as “20/20 vision or your money back” or “lifetime guarantee.” Of necessity, such statements contain fine print and initiate the doctor-patient relationship in a rather deceptive manner. Go elsewhere. You are not buying a car.

This is real surgery. Your surgeon should be well aware of the limits of LASIK and readily acknowledge the probability of complications in high risk patients.

Internet Research: Proceed with caution

Many leading LASIK surgeons have taken the extra effort to establish web sites that can detail their practice, qualifications, and success rates. This information is useful in your research. However, the web is also filled with inaccurate information. A small group of patients may voice concerns over complications. Keep in mind, that these may be the patients who had the procedure performed with older technology, before the Intralase and before wavefront-guided LASIK. Many of their concerns can be resolved with simple post-operative treatments, such as specific drops for your dry eyes, or wavefront-guided enhancement to improve night time vision. If you have a good rapport with your surgeon, you should be able to bring up your concerns to him or her directly and let them help you.

While you investigate, don't lose sight of the benefits: for most people, a lifetime of bad vision can be cured in fifteen minutes.

Custom LASIK has improved the eyesight of over a million people around the world. Your LASIK surgeon need not be your best friend, but you should have every confidence that he or she possesses the skill and experience necessary to apply the technique of Custom LASIK in a way that best serves your interests.

8
Initial Consultation

THE FIRST STEP IN YOUR CUSTOM LASIK PROCEDURE is the consultation which is important for several reasons. First, it must be determined whether you are a good candidate. Second, it is also vital for you to learn as much as you can about your options and have as many of your questions answered as possible.

The style of the initial consultation may vary between different surgeons. Some surgeons may not require you to be out of contact lenses prior to coming in. They will perform autorefraction to measure your prescription, topography to examine the shape of your cornea, and pachymetry to check the corneal thickness. Based on the results of these tests, they will determine if they can perform Custom LASIK for you. If not, they will recommend the best procedure. After you have been out of contacts for the recommended period of time, you will come in for your pre-procedural exam where a more thorough eye examination will be performed to get you ready for the procedure. With some laser systems, your pre-procedural exam can be done on the same day as your procedure. At this visit, a detailed eye examination is performed. Depending on the results of this examination, you may be asked to stay out of contact lenses longer and then come in again for another examination prior to your procedure.

Some patients may prefer to come in for a brief consultation first to simply find out if they can have Custom LASIK and not bother staying out of contacts if they can't have the procedure. If they can have the procedure, they can simply remove the contacts for the specific time prescribed to them rather than a generic length of time which may not even be necessary. Additionally, the shorter consultation is typically free, while there is usually a charge for the longer exam. If for some reason you are not a candidate, you may not want to incur the expense of a full examination.

The first step to Custom LASIK is to find out if you are an excellent candidate.

What to Expect During the Consultation

Required Tests

1) Meet the Counselor
    a) Share your interests
    b) Understand your specific needs
2) Watch an educational video about Custom LASIK
    a) Comprehend the technology and the procedure
3) History: It is important to disclose your full medical history when assessing whether Custom LASIK is the right procedure for you.
    a) Occupation – tailor the procedure to your individual needs
    b) Contact lens wear – contact type and extent of wear (daily wear, extended wear, gas permeable). Patients that use soft contacts should refrain from wear for 1-2 weeks and those that use gas permeable contacts should refrain from wear for 4-8 weeks
    c) Reading glasses – any problems
    d) Stability of vision
    e) History of glare or halos
    f) History of previous eye surgeries
    g) History of medical diseases, i.e., herpes simplex eye infection, rheumatoid arthritis, lupus, autoimmune disease and drug intake

h) Use of a pacemaker
i) History of migraine headaches
j) History of dry eyes
k) Familiarity with monovision for presbyopic patients

Autorefraction
Automated equipment that measures your prescription by projecting light to the back of your eye and measuring its shape when it comes out. Typically, this test is about 95% accurate in measuring your prescription enough to determine what procedure is best for you. If your autorefraction result is marginal, then the doctor may perform manual refraction at the phoropter.

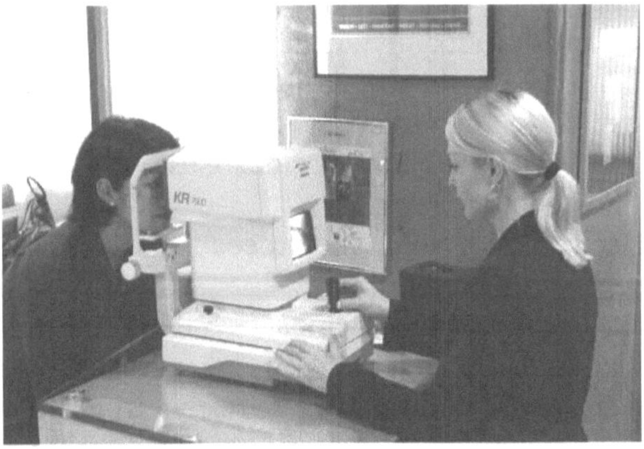

Autorefraction is often the first step in your Custom LASIK process

Topography
Corneal mapping to determine the smoothness and symmetry of your cornea. The importance of topography is primarily to identify patients with a bulging cornea, i.e., keretoconus – a contraindication for surgery. There are different types of topography systems, however, the standard of this care at

this time is utilizing a system called the orbscan or better yet, the pentacam.

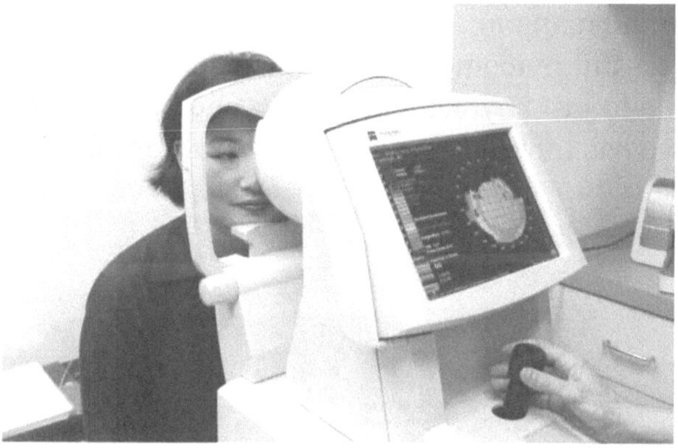

Corneal topography (elevation map) is performed to evaluate the corneal surface

Pachymetry

Ultrasound measurement of your corneal thickness. Average corneal thickness is between 500 and 600 microns. The thickness, however, may vary by as much as 30 microns from exam to exam. If your corneal thickness is marginal, it should be rechecked once you are out of contact lenses for 2 weeks. Some surgeons refrain from performing Custom LASIK in cases less than 500 microns to avoid weakening the cornea, i.e., ectasia.

Tonometry

Your eye pressure will be measured by a digital device to rule out glaucoma.

Wavefront Mapping

You will be seated in front of the wavefront aberrometer and asked to look at the red light. The ophthalmic technician will perform the mapping. The mapping step is very important to the successful outcome of your procedure and should not be delegated to just anyone. A highly trained team member with extensive background in eye care is ideal for this step.

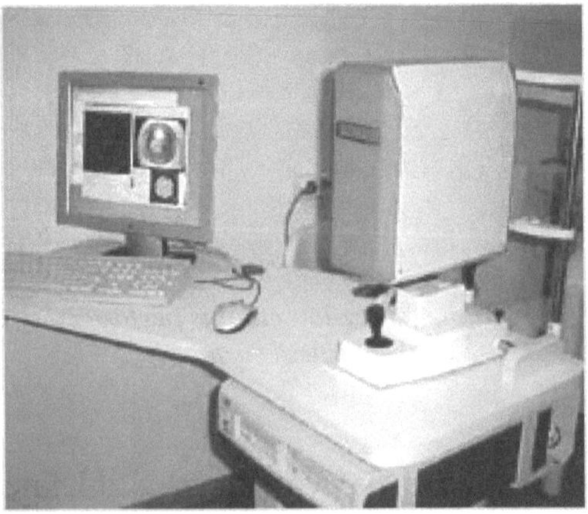

The aberrometer captures the unique imperfections of your vision.

Manifest Refraction

Your prescription will be measured with technology called the phoropter. Different lenses will be dialed in and you will be asked to choose which is better, "one" of "two" or "both." Do not worry about making the "right choice." Your vision will be tested in different ways to make sure that the measurements are consistent.

Pupil Size

Pupil size will be measured with infrared pupillometer to determine its size in the dark. One should make sure that the laser treatment zone is larger than the pupil size in the dark state to avoid halos and glare at night.

Slit lamp examination

Utilizing the magnifying equipment, the surgeon will examine your eyelids, conjunctiva, tear film, corneal health, and ensure that you do not have a cataract. Following ruling out any lid infections, conjunctivitis and corneal degeneration, a thorough assessment of the eye for dryness is completed, i.e., shirmer tear test, tear meniscus, tear breakup time and rose bengal test. Dry eyes need to be treated aggressively prior to the procedure, preferably by placing tear drops frequently, utililization of Restasis drops that potentiate tear productivity or placement of tear duct plug.

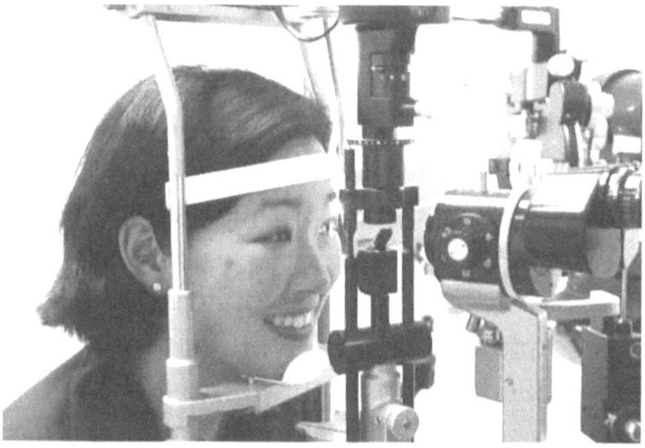

Slit lamp examination is performed to evaluate the tear film and the health of your eyes

Eye Dilation and Cycloplegic Refraction

An eye drop will be used to dilate your pupils and to temporarily immobilize your lens so that it can relax and stop accommodating. Pupil dilation allows the doctor to examine the back of your eye – your retina and optic nerve. Generally, the eye dilation should last about 4 hours. Occasionally, especially in younger patients, a strong dilating drop may be used. The effect of this drop may last into the following day.

Discussion

Once all the information is gathered, you will have a discussion with your surgeon. The surgeon will review your medical and vision history. It is important for your doctor to know everything about your medical history as certain systemic diseases such as rheumatoid arthritis, lupus, and other autoimmune diseases are a contraindication. Certain healing disorders, diabetes, a cardiac pacemaker, and a current or planned pregnancy may need special consideration. The ocular history will include questions about previous contact lens wear and eye disease. The doctor will want to know if you have dry eye and/or if you've had a history of recurrent erosions or basement membrane disease.

Another eye disease that the doctor must be aware of is *herpes simplex* on the eyes as well as potential kerotoconus. The doctor will explain to you that diseases such as glaucoma or diabetes will not preclude you from having the procedure, but they must be identified and controlled. It is important for you to notify the doctor during the consultation of any ongoing changes or problems with your vision. If you have a significant cataract, you should not undergo LASIK vision correction.

Please be prepared to let the surgeon know your medications and allergies.

To be a candidate for Custom LASIK, you must meet the following requirements:

- Be over eighteen years of age
- Myopia up to –12.00 diopters or hyperopia up to +6.00 diopters, with or without astigmatism (up to 3.00 diopters).
- Stable vision for at least a year.
- Be free from certain diseases of the cornea, lens, and retina.
- Not pregnant or nursing

The following are NOT CONTRAINDICATIONS to laser vision correction, but need to be discussed with your surgeon:

- History of glaucoma, uveitis, certain corneal irregularities
- Previous eye surgery including radial keratotomy (RK), PRK, lens surgery, cataract surgery, corneal transplant
- Diabetes
- Advanced age

Informed Consent

Prior to your surgery date you will have the opportunity to read and understand the informed consent. Any remaining questions that you may have about the healing process and what to expect during and after the procedure should be addressed prior to surgery.

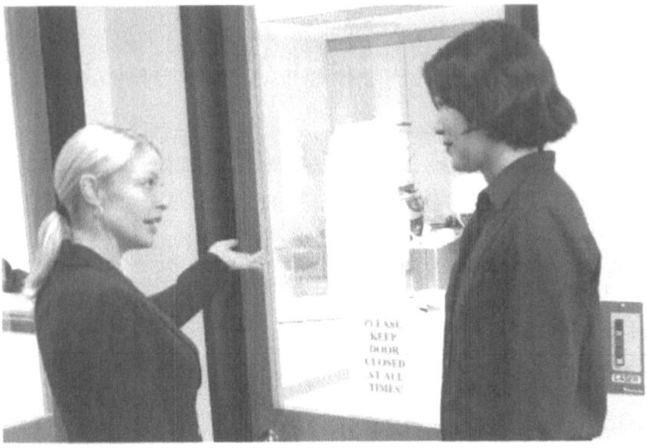

Patient reviews the steps of the Custom LASIK procedure

Patients over age 40 that are interested in preserving their reading vision may experience monovision, where one eye is corrected for distance and the other for reading. Such a combination can be demonstrated with a temporary contact lens fitting to simulate the outcome.

Tour of the facility

Of all the concerns that people face considering refractive surgery, fear of the unknown is perhaps the greatest. By touring the facility, seeing where you will have your procedure, you can be assured that you are in good hands and all will be taken care of for you.

9

The Day of Your Custom LASIK Procedure

ON THE DAY OF YOUR PROCEDURE, you should arrive at the laser center as rested and relaxed as possible. You should probably allow about a two hour stay at the laser center. This may vary from center to center. You will need to arrange transportation for the day of the procedure. Wear comfortable clothing. Do not wear makeup, perfume, or cologne on the day of your laser surgery. These things may interfere with the cleanliness of the procedure and the function of the excimer laser. Likewise, do not wear your hair in a bun. Your head needs to lie flat during the procedure, and the bun will cause your head to be unstable and uncomfortable.

Contact lenses must be removed from the operate eye as recommended by your surgeon. However, as a rule of thumb, soft contact lenses need to be out for 2 weeks, gas permeable hard lenses 4 weeks, and toric contact lenses 3 weeks. It is essential that your eye be in its most natural state at the time of surgery. You will be given a consent form to read and sign. The majority of surgeons will meet you at that time to review the date, set the plan and demarcate your astigmatism to offset any cycloversion movement during surgery.

Prepping for Custom LASIK

With Custom LASIK, a mild oral sedative may be administered before the procedure begins. During the procedure, your surgeon and the team will be talking to you. They will talk you through the entire procedure; you will know at all times what to expect.

Because Custom LASIK is surgical in nature, sterile surgical conditions must be maintained. You will be given an antibiotic drop, a nonsteroidal anti-inflammatory drop, and an anesthetic drop to improve comfort. You will also be given a surgical cap to wear. While the drops begin to work, the area around your eyes will be cleaned with a betadine disinfectant.

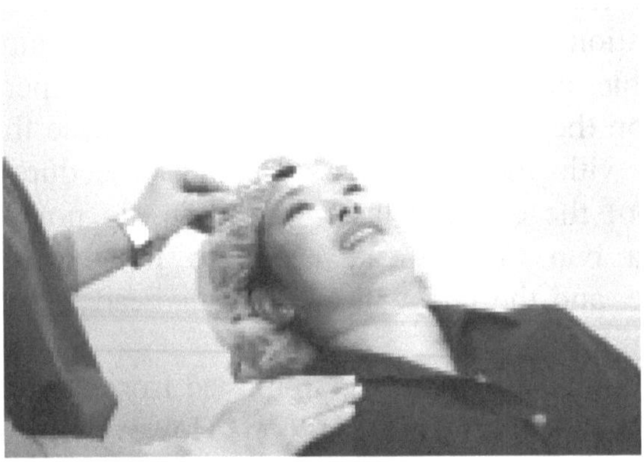

Patient is lying down in preparation for the procedure.

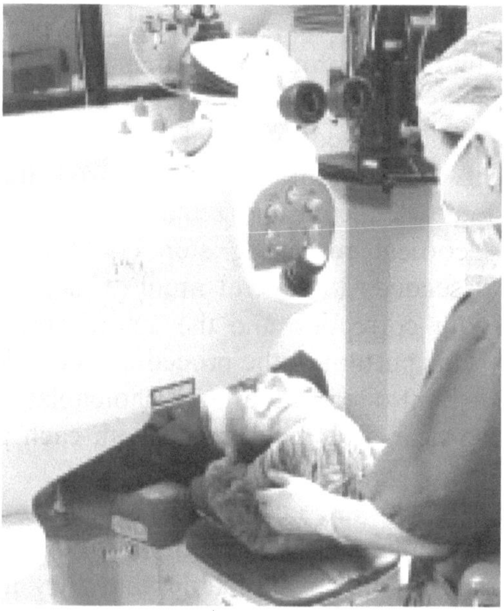

The patient is positioned under the Intralase in preparation for formation of the corneal flap.

The Procedure:

Step 1: Creating the Corneal Flap

You will be positioned properly under the laser microscope and the fellow eye will be covered. Additional anesthetic drops will be placed in the operative eye. During the process of creating the corneal flap, you will feel pressure sensation and the lights go dark. Depending on the surgeon's preference, he may utilize a microkeratome or the Intralase in making a flap.

Step 2: Custom Corneal Reshaping

The superficial layer will be unfolded and your vision will get blurry. You will be asked to fix your vision on a red flashing light, which may appear slightly orange or yellow in color. The laser part of the procedure is then performed, and is regulated by the pre-programmed mapping.

Advanced laser systems are also equipped with a high speed computerized eye tracker that helps to enhance the treatment by providing the precise registration of the laser beam to create the customized ablation surface.

This corneal reshaping step could take anywhere from several seconds to several minutes, depending on the amount of your correction and the amount of higher order aberrations. This portion of the procedure is painless, but you may notice a faint odor as the laser photoablation proceeds. You will also hear a clicking sound with each pulse of the laser.

Your eyes are continually making very fine “saccadic” movements that are jumping movements. These movements are simply unavoidable since, try as you may, you will be unable to control them. As your eye moves, it will appear as though the fixation light is moving. Keep following the red fixation target light and you will be fine. The tracking system in the advanced lasers assists the surgery by scanning the eye thousands of times per second and by making computer micro-adjustments many times per second to reposition the pinpoint laser beam between pulses of light. This technology tracks the very smallest and quickest movements of your eye throughout this phase of the treatment.

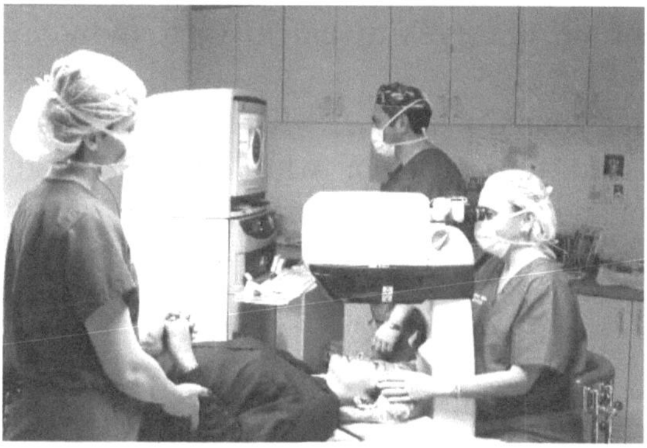

The patient has been prepped and is ready for corneal reshaping with the excimer laser.

The excimer laser is designed to use an ultra-small beam of cool laser light — one that is less than a millimeter wide, a good deal smaller than the thickness of a single hair. Using high speed computer control, the excimer laser moves this tiny beam of rapid light across the surface of the cornea in a tiny, non-sequential and overlapping pattern. The result is a smooth customized corneal shape that gives a fast visual recovery and individualized correction.

At the completion of the ablation, the superficial corneal layer is placed back into its original position and your vision will clear somewhat. There is a slight waiting period for the eye to create a natural vacuum to hold the flap down. The cornea has the unique ability to seal itself naturally back into place resulting in a complete and smooth replacement. This simply indicates how marvelous the human eye is at adaptation.

After the drying is completed, the lid retractor is removed and you are able to blink normally. In some patients, the surgeon may place a clear non-prescription contact lens on the eyes to aid in their individual healing process.

After your Custom LASIK surgery is completed, you will be asked to remain a while in the surgicenter for observation and postoperative instructions.

10 Postoperative Care after Custom LASIK

ONCE YOUR PROCEDURE IS COMPLETED, antibiotic drops will be instilled and clear plastic shields will be placed over your eyes to protect them. You will then be instructed to go home and take a nap. You will be asked to keep your eyes closed, typically for four hours, to allow adequate initial healing. Because your vision will be blurry and you have received a sedative, you will need to have someone drive you.

Typically, you will be instructed to wear the clear plastic shields over your eyes for one to three nights. These prevent accidental trauma to the corneal surface during the healing period should you inadvertently bump your eye.

Before you go home to rest, your surgeon may also give you something to help you sleep, for this is the best way to keep your eyes closed for the first few hours. Following LASIK surgery, you may experience some burning or discomfort, which may last a couple of hours. Patients describe the discomfort as a "sandy feeling" or liken it to having a dirty contact lens in their eye.

With LASIK, this discomfort typically subsides with sleep and is usually gone by the next day. Tylenol®, ibuprofen, or similar over the counter pain medications are usually adequate to keep you comfortable.

You will also be given antibiotic eye drops, anti-inflammatory eye drops, and lubricant eye drops to promote healing. It is common for the eyes to feel somewhat dry, and the lubricant drops (also called "artificial tears") may be used frequently.

Immediately after the surgery, you can expect your vision to be fairly blurry. It may look as though you are looking through a glass of water or fog. With Custom LASIK there is usually a dramatic improvement in vision in the first twenty four hours.

Guidelines for Healing

Follow these guidelines to promote safe and rapid healing:

- Rest and sleep aid recovery.
- Particularly in dry climates, apply nonpreserved lubricant eye drops very frequently. This encourages rapid recovery and enhances comfort. (Some patients may need these drops every hour the first few days, every couple of hours the first week, and at least four times daily for the first three months.)
- Sensitivity to light is normal and will improve. Wear good ultraviolet-protecting sunglasses.
- Avoid rubbing your eyes and squeezing your eye lids, especially during the first twenty four hours after surgery. You can rub your eyes gently two weeks after surgery.
- Avoid swimming and hot tubs for one week.
- Showers and baths are fine, but try to avoid getting water and shampoo directly into your eyes for at least two weeks.
- Cardiovascular exercise is fine the next day. You can resume heavy weight lifting in a week. Avoid getting sweat in your eyes during the first week.
- Avoid dusty or smoky environments immediately after surgery.
- Avoid eye makeup for one week.

- It is a good idea to plan on not driving until you feel your vision has improved. You may drive as soon as you are visually comfortable. This may be the next day or may take a few days.

Postoperative Follow-up Schedule

When you leave the laser center, you will be given complete instructions to follow, including a postoperative appointment schedule. Here is a typical postoperative appointment schedule:

Purpose of Appointment	**Time**
To ensure that there is no evidence of infection, that the surface is healing properly, and to remove the bandage contact lens (if one was used)	1 day
To ensure that your eye is healing properly	1 wk., 1 mo.
To measure your visual progress and to consider enhancement treatment (if necessary)	3–6 months
To measure the stability of your result, check your eye pressure, and assess your general eye health	12 months

The Custom LASIK Recovery Cycle

Your vision improves quickly after Custom LASIK, and many patients feel comfortable enough to drive in one to two days. The superficial corneal layer is relatively adhered in one week, but it is advisable not to rub your eyes vigorously for one month.

For the first three to seven days after your surgery, you will be using medicated eye drops. It is generally advisable to continue using lubricant drops for the better part of the first month after your procedure. Well lubricated eyes heal better, maintain better visual stability, and are more comfortable. These drops are available over the counter. Your doctor can advise you on which drops are best for you.

The return of visual stability after Custom LASIK varies for each patient. For some, stability can be achieved in as few as one to two weeks; for others, stability may take up to six months. As a rule, vision will improve in three hours, more in three days, three weeks, and even in three months. Generally, during the course of the first month, there is gradual improvement in good vision following Custom LASIK. You can also expect a reduction in nighttime halos and some return of near vision in patients over forty.

It is important that you keep your postoperative appointments as your drop regimen may be altered. Also, the doctor needs to monitor your eye pressure if you are on postoperative steroids for two weeks or longer. Be sure to keep your follow-up appointments.

Most patients enjoy good functional vision during the first month. Fluctuations in your vision are common during the first two to three weeks, especially for higher visual corrections. Patients undergoing hyperopic Custom LASIK (farsightedness treatment), especially in the higher ranges (+3.00 to +6.00 diopters), will notice that their visual recovery is typically slower compared to patients having myopic LASIK (nearsightedness treatment). After farsightedness treatment, patients often notice that their near vision is better than their distance vision. This is quite common, and their distance vision will continue to improve during the first month.

Some patients may feel more comfortable with a thin pair of glasses to assist them with more critical distance vision activities, such as night driving or attending a play and trying to see the expressions on the actors' faces. Patients over forty years of age may require a thin pair of reading glasses.

While many patients notice halos around lights or ghosting of images at night, these symptoms tend to diminish substantially over the first month.

Patients with a history of dry eyes, or who use the computer, read for long hours, drive long distances, or live in low-humidity climates may notice some minor discomfort and blurring of their vision, particularly toward the end of the day. This is usually related to dryness of the surface of the eye. The frequent use of lubricant drops and a conscious effort by the patient to blink more during these activities will help significantly.

With Custom LASIK, your vision usually becomes stable within three to six months. Once your vision is stable, your treatment is permanent. You now have less dependence on, and maybe complete freedom from glasses and contact lenses.

11
Patient Results with Custom LASIK

THE DECISION TO UNDERGO CUSTOM LASIK refractive surgery is based on either vocation, convenience, or safety reasons, which makes it an elective procedure rather than a medical necessity. The decision to have the surgery is completely up to you, unless the surgeon determines that you, for medical or other reasons, need to have the procedure. For example, if you keep getting corneal infections or abrasions with contact lenses, Custom LASIK may be a safer option for you.

There are many ways to present patient outcomes after refractive surgery, and the difference in numbers can be confusing. Some doctors may talk about the percentage of patients who achieve 20/20 vision after the first treatment, while others may present data on the number of patients who achieve 20/40 vision. Still others may discuss their results based on patients who have had enhancement procedures (if necessary). What are the important numbers and how can you interpret these outcomes?

First of all, to drive legally without glasses you need to have 20/40 vision. This is an important number; however, it is also important to know your chance of achieving 20/20 or better vision without glasses. Additionally, it is important to know the likelihood that you will need an enhancement (re-treatment) procedure. These numbers depend on your initial prescription and are also surgeon dependent. Patients with higher degrees of nearsightedness, farsightedness, or astigmatism have a higher likelihood of needing an enhancement procedure. Surgeons who are reluctant to do an enhancement or have minimum visual acuity cut off requirements for enhancement will have a lower enhancement rate. Surgeons who are comfortable doing small touch ups, are more likely to fine tune patients' vision with enhancement.

Keep in mind that even the patients who do not achieve 20/20 vision without glasses are usually happy. They can do most things, including drive a car, without any correction. And when it is absolutely necessary for them to see 20/20, they can use a thin pair of glasses to do so.

With Custom LASIK, an experienced surgeon can give you great vision. In the FDA studies, over 90% of patients achieved 20/20 or better vision without glasses or contact lenses.

In the U.S. Navy studies, patients saw better with Custom LASIK compared to conventional laser treatments. Not only did they have better visual acuity, but also, better contrast sensitivity and better ability to see well in dim light.

Nighttime vision is significantly better with Custom LASIK. The chance of glare and halos is reduced. In fact, the chance of you having fewer imperfections in your vision than you had with glasses or contact lenses is five times better with the wavefront-guided Custom LASIK than with the conventional procedure.

Medical studies and scientific data may provide compelling evidence in support of having Custom LASIK vision correction performed. Nevertheless, the most convincing testimonies come from the many patients who provide firsthand accounts of their procedures that resulted in much improved vision and a better quality of life.

For the benefit of potential patients who are considering LASIK surgery, comments from several individuals are given in the following pages.

"I want to give all of you a heartfelt thanks. I put off having LASIK for years – mostly out of fear. I know the importance of having an exceptional surgeon, especially considering I am married to an ophthalmologist. I also know the importance of the surgeon using the safest technology. My new vision is nothing short of miraculous. I can actually see what I'm doing when I put make up on. We went to Yosemite a few weeks ago and I could see individual pine needles on the trees at quite a far distance. It is as if I'm looking at a whole, new, crisp world. Thank you for dramatically improving the life of your patients. What a phenomenal work!" — Carly V.

"I woke up this morning, as I do every morning, thrilled and amazed at how clearly I can see the numbers on the clock across the room. Nine months ago, I did not have this luxury. Thanks to your superb skill and expertise performing my Custom LASIK procedure, this is just one of the many daily benefits I continue to enjoy!

As an optometrist, I am very informed about the many refractive procedures and practices made available to my patients today. I can say that you have provided me, as well as many of my patients, the very best treatment and the best results. Throughout the entire process, I felt well informed, relaxed, and secure. Because of the great trust and respect and my great results, I have sent you my family for Custom LASIK. My three brothers all had the same fantastic experiences, and the three sisters are next!"
— Dr. Manny N.

"My new eyes work! I ran the Dipsea race last Sunday with my new eyes! No problems running up and over Mt. Tam, playing tennis, swimming in the pool – this is a new and wonderful chapter in my life! Many thanks for the great gift you gave me. Every morning is a reminder of the miracle of clear sight!" — Kevin E.

"I'd like to thank you for performing Custom LASIK on me earlier this month. It is a life changing experience for me to be able to do simple things minus my contacts or glasses such as swimming or seeing what I'm actually doing in the shower early in the morning!

It was your experience and the latest technology that prompted me to do the surgery at this point in time. Both the wavefront technology and the Intralase laser are what convinced me that side effects would be minimal to someone with moderate myopia. Before this technology, my concerns, as an eye care provider, were halos at night and complications with the microkeratome blade. All of which is critical to scientific minds like you and me.

It is the high success rate of the wavefront that convinced me that Custom LASIK would be a possibility to me. Your integration of the Intralase into your practice was the thing that prompted me to do the surgery at this time. The complications with the laser rather than a blade are reduced to a minimum, which is what has increased the safety factor for me to proceed with the procedure.

Your willingness to explore, study, and then use the new technology (if needed) is what implores me to recommend all my patients to see you when they consider refractive surgery. I know that you will honestly tell them if they are or are not a good candidate for laser surgery, and which procedure will benefit them the most."
— Dr. Michelle B.

12
Possible Risks with Custom LASIK

IN ORDER TO MAKE A DECISION as to whether Custom LASIK vision correction surgery is a good alternative for you, it is important to understand the potential risks. If performed by an experienced surgeon, the risks are low—it is one of the safest surgeries performed today.

The following are several factors that enter into whether or not the proper correction is achieved.

Unrealistic expectations

It is wise for those who undergo Custom LASIK to be fully informed and carefully assess their expectations. As a patient, your job is to understand exactly what the procedure can and cannot do. This is where communication with your doctor is essential. Your doctor should understand all of your expectations, and then explain what is realistic and what is not. Although this procedure is one of the most successful in all of medicine, even the most skilled and experienced surgeon cannot promise that you will have 20/20 vision correction.

With Custom LASIK a skilled surgeon can significantly reduce your dependence on glasses and contact lenses.

Dry Eye

Some patients experience a "grittiness" following Custom LASIK. This condition usually tends to resolve itself over the first one to three months. In the meantime, adequate application of the lubricating eye drops will often alleviate the symptoms.

It is important that your doctor evaluate you for dry eyes prior to the Custom LASIK procedure. If dryness exists prior to surgery, or if dry eye symptoms persist after surgery despite the frequent use of artificial tears, your doctor may recommend blocking your tear drainage canals with punctual plugs. This brief, painless procedure prevents your natural tears from draining away so quickly and results in improved lubrication of the surface of the eye. The use of Restasis eye drops has been proven to potentiate an increase in tear production.

Corneal Abrasion

Infrequently, one may develop a small corneal abrasion during Custom LASIK. Despite excellent surgical technique and an adequately moistened eye, a small breakdown in the epithelial surface may develop as the flap is made. Corneal abrasions are noted more so with the microkeratome rather than Intralase. This occurs in approximately 3% of Custom LASIK procedures because the surface cells do not adhere well. The medical term for this is epithelial basement membrane disorder. Unfortunately, doctors cannot always detect this preoperatively. A very thin bandage contact lens may be placed on the eye if this occurs to improve comfort and promote healing. The bandage contact lens is usually removed within the next few days. Fortunately, the epithelium grows back rapidly, usually healing within one to three days.

Night Glare and Halos

It is not uncommon for nearsighted patients who wear glasses or contacts to have symptoms of glare or see halos or starbursts at night. This is due to having longer eyes than normal sighted patients. Thus, at night in a nearsighted patient when the pupil dilates, peripheral light rays are scattered more before reaching the retina. It is this scattering that results in glare and halos.

With Custom LASIK, the chance of glare and halos is reduced significantly. Some patients with large dilating pupils and large corrections may not be optimal candidates for Custom LASIK, as their risk of glare and halos may be higher. Special laser programs that allow larger treatment zones can help reduce the chance of these problems. Your surgeon will optimize the size of the treatment zone based on how widely your pupils dilate at night.

Inflammation

A mild inflammation, called diffuse lamellar keratitis can sometimes occur under the flap. Although most patients have no symptoms, some may experience light sensitivity. The condition is typically treated with anti-inflammatory drops. Prevention requires maintaining meticulous surgical technique. After your procedure, you are routinely given the anti-inflammatory steroid drops to use for a week or so. These drops help prevent inflammation as well.

Corneal Flap Risks

With the advent of Intralase FS laser technology, the safety of the procedure increased significantly. In very rare instances the flap may show some straie (microscopic fold) which rarely interferes with vision. However, with time, this dissipates. Patients may worry about displacement of the flap. Nevertheless, this is extremely rare and is manageable.

Epithelial Ingrowth

Rarely, some of the corneal surface cells (epithelium) may get trapped beneath the flap. These cells typically do not create any problem, but occasionally they can cause mild blurriness or irritation. This problem can be easily identified and treated by gently lifting the flap and removing the trapped epithelial cells.

Undercorrection and Overcorrection

For a degree of nearsightedness or farsightedness, the amount of laser applied to a patient's cornea is based on the average person's response to the laser. However, individuals are different and may respond differently. Usually, this difference in response is not visually significant, but sometimes an undercorrection or overcorrection will occur.

Undercorrection is more common than overcorrection. A slight undercorrection will not seriously affect your vision and may be desirable following a nearsighted treatment in patients over forty to help with reading vision. Significant undercorrections may require an enhancement procedure (which is usually included in the original Custom LASIK fee).

Undercorrection and overcorrection are eliminated by surgeons using consistent technique and constantly analyzing their outcomes. Your doctor should keep an up to date database of procedures and be able to tell you what the likelihood is of needing retreatment.

The excimer laser comes from the factory with standard recommended settings. By fine tuning the factory treatment parameters, the surgeon minimizes the chance of undercorrection.

An initial overcorrection following a myopic treatment may occur and usually corrects itself within a few months. Following a hyperopic treatment, an overcorrection will make you temporarily nearsighted, making your distance vision somewhat blurry and your near vision rather good. These temporary undercorrections and overcorrections can be managed with glasses until they resolve. The number of overcorrections is fewer than that of undercorrections. The incidence of undercorrections and overcorrections in the best hands should not exceed 5%.

Enhancement procedures

Medically indicated enhancements are generally performed at least three months after the original treatment at no additional cost to the patient. The original flap created during the Custom LASIK procedure is lifted with a specially designed instrument. There is usually no need to cut a new flap; thus, the risks associated with creating the flap originally are not a factor in re-treatment. Postoperative healing is normally faster than following the original procedure and the vision stabilizes quicker, because corrections are typically smaller. Your doctor can decide on the frequency of additional enhancements.

Decrease of Best Corrected Vision

A small number of patients may experience a slight decrease of visual sharpness following Custom LASIK vision correction. This means that even with glasses, you may lose some of the crispness and clarity of your vision. This can be due to irregular healing and usually improves over time. Careful surgical technique and good follow-up care help minimize the incidence of this problem. The incidence of this occurrence is less than 1% and it typically improves over time.

Infection

Although infection is the most feared complication, it is extremely rare. As with any surgery, it is avoided through sterile surgical technique and the use of prophylactic antibiotic drops postoperatively. If it does occur, it manifests itself in the first twenty-four to seventy-two hours after treatment. That is why it is important for you to go to all of your follow-up visits, even if everything seems to be fine. However, in an exceedingly rare instance of an infection, it can be treated with antibiotic drops.

Regression

Regression refers to the tendency of the vision to drift back slightly toward its original prescription. This occurs more commonly in patients with higher amounts of myopia, hyperopia, or astigmatism. In myopic and hyperopic patients, there may an inclination for very negligible change in the prescription with age. This change may marginally impact the quality of vision. An enhancement can be performed to help with these changes.

If regression makes your vision blurry, an enhancement procedure may be performed to "tune up" the original treatment. Enhancements for regression are usually performed anywhere from one year to five years following the original procedure to allow time for the patient's new refraction to stabilize. In some cases, glasses for night driving may be all that is needed.

Summary

Custom LASIK is the procedure of choice for virtually all but the most extreme myopic and hyperopic patients. In addition, most degrees of astigmatism can be treated. It is a very precise procedure and allows for accurate enhancements when needed.

From the information presented above, you can see that while refractive surgery is an exciting new procedure, it is not for everyone. It is important to understand the natural limitations of the eye (such as presbyopia) and any specific conditions that you may have. It should not be thought of as a guarantee to eliminate one's need for glasses. Rather, it should be thought of as a way to dramatically reduce one's dependency on glasses and contact lenses.

13
Questions and Answers

Q. Am I too old to have Custom LASIK?
A. There is no upper age limit to Custom LASIK. Patients in their 90's have had Custom LASIK eye surgery. Your doctor will examine both eyes thoroughly. If your eyes are healthy, you should definitely consider this procedure to help you see better without glasses or contact lenses.

Q. Am I too young to have Custom LASIK?
A. The lower age limit recommended by the FDA is 18 years old. Your vision has to be stable (i.e. your prescription within 0.5 diopters) for at least a year and your eyes must be healthy. Younger patients often undergo Custom LASIK to help them in sports, to avoid wearing contact lenses during extended studying times, and prior to serving military duty or starting police or firefighter work.

Q. Can I fly after LASIK?
A. Certainly. The cabin air is pressurized, so it is similar to being on the ground. However, the environment is very dry, so you will need to use lubricating drops every hour. Some patients may be concerned traveling the second day following the procedure. Nonetheless, you can even fly the day after your Custom LASIK procedure.

Q. Can I scuba dive after Custom LASIK?
A. Certainly. You should wait at least three weeks before getting into the water. After that, you can scuba dive. A recent scientific study published in the Journal of Cataract and Refractive Surgery evaluated the safety of scuba diving as deep as 100 ft on Navy SEALS who had LASIK. Scuba diving after LASIK had no effect on the eyes at all and was found to be safe.

Q. Can I mountain climb after Custom LASIK?
A. You certainly can! There should be no effect on vision at any elevation.

Q. Will my night vision get worse after Custom LASIK?
A. Many studies have shown that night vision remains excellent after Custom LASIK. In many patients, it's even better than their night vision with their glasses or contact lenses. As the eyes heal, especially during the first month after the procedure, some patients may experience glare at night. This goes away with time. If it doesn't, an enhancement may help. Custom LASIK, with advanced wavefront technology, improves the quality of vision both day and night.

Q. My eyes already feel dry with contact lenses. Does it preclude me from having LASIK? Will my eyes feel dryer after LASIK?
A. Contact lenses may prevent normal tear film circulation and many people actually experience the sensation of dryness while wearing contact lenses. This doesn't necessarily mean that your eyes are actually dry. Typically, your doctor will ask you to stay out of contact lenses for at least a week before the preoperative exam to let your tear film stabilize. Your eyes will then be tested specifically for

dryness. Even if you do have some dryness, it doesn't necessarily preclude you from having Custom LASIK. Your doctor may give you drops or place plugs in your tear ducts to help your eyes accumulate more tears. Also, studies have shown that with Intralase, the incidence of dryness is reduced significantly, compared to the mechanical microkeratome.

Q. If I have Custom LASIK now, will I need to get it done again in the future?
A. Custom LASIK is a permanent correction. Your prescription should not "go back" or "reverse." Between three and six months after the procedure, your doctor will check your vision. If you have a little bit of nearsightedness, farsightedness, or astigmatism causing blurry vision, you may have an enhancement to eliminate it if medically safe. Only about 5% of patients need an enhancement. Your vision should stay stable after the enhancement.

Q. If a patient had conventional LASIK in the past, can that person qualify for Custom Wavefront LASIK?
A. Patients who have already undergone a LASIK procedure can be evaluated with the wavefront scan system. An enhancement procedure can be performed with Custom Wavefront technology if higher-order aberrations are present.

Q. Will LASIK accelerate my need for reading glasses?
A. The need for reading glasses, also called presbyopia, develops as the lens inside the eye gets harder and can't accommodate anymore to focus on near objects. This typically happens in our 40's. With Custom LASIK, the surgeon will correct the shape of your cornea to improve your distance vision. The lens changes will happen

regardless of whether you have LASIK or not. LASIK will not speed up presbyopia. Most people will still need to wear reading glasses in their 40's.

Q. What is Presbyopia?

A. It is a vision condition caused by loss of flexibility of the crystalline lens that makes it difficult for one to focus on close objects, i.e., reading. It affects most people in their mid-forties. It is easily recognized when a patient holds reading material at arms length. To correct presbyopia your doctor may prescribe reading glasses, bifocals or contact lenses.

Q. Can Custom LASIK correct presbyopia?

A. Custom LASIK cannot correct presbyopia. However, there have been some modifications of the laser treatment to provide presbyopic patients with Monovision as a solution.

Q. How does Monovision work?

A. Your doctor will correct your dominant eye for distance vision and your non-dominant eye for reading. Eye dominance is analogous to right or left handedness. Your doctor typically will identify the dominant eye. Because monovision can affect your optimum depth perception, it is recommended that your doctor place a contact lens in your eye to simulate your post operative vision. If one has any hesitation whatsoever, surgery should be put on hold until comfort level is attained with monovision contact lenses.

Q. Should I have Custom LASIK done now or should I wait for new technologies?

A. An experienced surgeon using current state-of-the-art technology can give his or her patients outstanding vision without contacts or glasses, both day and night. If your eyes are healthy and your prescription is within the range of the currently available technology, you should experience excellent vision after the procedure. It would be a pity to deny yourself that excellent vision while you are waiting for "the next best thing." However, if your prescription is outside the range of currently available technology or is at the upper most limit of it, it would be reasonable to wait until the technology allows your surgeon to offer an excellent outcome.

Conclusion

CUSTOM LASIK IS THE MOST IMPORTANT ADVANCE in the sub-specialty of refractive surgery. Custom LASIK has improved the outcomes and stability of refractive surgery. It has gained widespread acceptance in the field of ophthalmology and optometry, and with the general public in the past two years.

What does the future hold? Currently in the United States, myopia, hyperopia, and astigmatism have all been approved for treatment.

Refractive surgery is becoming more and more commonplace. Some speculate that children will get their braces at twelve, their driver's license at sixteen, and their refractive surgery at eighteen.

Appendix History—Timeline of Refractive Surgery

THE STUDY OF VISUAL PROBLEMS (refractive errors) began in the early sixteenth century when Leonardo da Vinci contemplated the possible source of visual disturbances. A little later, in 1619, Scheiner measured the anterior surface of the cornea. His discoveries are still used by ophthalmologists today who recognize that refractive surgery often depends on changing the cornea's anterior contour. Even lens removal as a means of correcting high degrees of myopia was discussed by Boerhaave in 1746. But real progress in the field of vision correction was constrained until a better understanding of how the eye functions was acquired.

Johannes E. Purkinje observed in 1823 that images form on optical surfaces when they reflect external light. His observations led to the development of the Purkinje principles and the four Purkinje images. From these developments our modern day understanding of keratometry (measuring the curvature of the cornea) and theories of visual accommodation began to grow.

Several decades later came the advent of topical (eye drop) anesthesia, which led to cataract surgery after the Civil War. In 1867, with the development of the keratometer (an instrument for measuring the curvature of the cornea), surgeons could measure astigmatism following cataract surgery.

In 1869 Snellen (after whom the vision charts of today are named) proposed using incisions across the steep meridian of the cornea to flatten it and treat astigmatism. However, twenty-one years would pass before anyone (Galezowski) would actually attempt to flatten the corneal contour (albeit unsuccessfully).

Trials and Experimentation

Not long after a successful cataract surgery technique was developed by van Graefe in the 1850s, ophthalmologists everywhere began to recognize the impact of corneal shape on astigmatism. In 1895 Faber performed a full thickness corneal incision to decrease naturally occurring astigmatism in a nineteen year old patient, thus enabling him to pass his vision test for entrance into the Royal Military Academy. But all of these efforts were focused on astigmatism; no one looked beyond astigmatism to myopia or hyperopia. It soon became apparent that a better understanding of the principles of keratotomy (the making of incisions in the cornea) was needed before any further progress could be made.

It was about this time that a Dutch physician, Leendert Jan Lans (working at the time on his doctoral degree), began to systematically study and define the principles of keratotomy. So fundamental and comprehensive was his research that it soon became the standard of refractive surgery. He practiced and promoted the principles of corneal flattening that could be achieved by incisions made on the anterior surface of the cornea. By varying the number, direction, and shape of the incisions, Lans could manipulate the effects and tailor the visual correction.

In addition to surgical techniques, there were non-surgical attempts at reducing myopia by manipulating the shape of the eye. One remedy was an eye cup with a spring-powered mallet designed to flatten the cornea; another was a firm rubber band used to flatten it. But these were techniques that failed to result in any significant degree of visual correction.

With the exception of the work performed by Lans, 1885 to 1939 was principally a time of trial and error for refractive surgery. Nevertheless, the successes and failures of this period helped determine which refractive procedures worked and which did not.

Modern Refractive Surgery

In 1936 Tsutomu Sato observed a flattening of the cornea in patients who had sustained traumatic injury to the eyes. The corneas of these patients were irregular and abnormally steep (keratoconus) but flattened after episodes of corneal swelling. His work led numerous scientists to establish the value of radial keratotomy, built upon the principles outlined by Lans nearly half a century earlier and applied to the treatment of keratoconus corneas. Sato brought anterior and posterior keratotomy to clinical practice in hundreds of patients and reported his results in the early 1940s. Other ophthalmic surgeons subsequently used his technique and obtained similar results.

Sato also applied his posterior keratotomy technique to the correction of astigmatism; this technique involved the disruption of the corneal endothelium, the internal cells on the backside of the cornea. Unfortunately, the role of the corneal endothelium in maintaining corneal thickness and clarity was not fully understood in Sato's time, and the subsequent development of corneal swelling in the majority of his patients who received this treatment went undetected until after his death.

In 1948 Ridley, a physician to Royal Air Force pilots in World War II noted that pilots whose eyes harbored slivers of Perspex (cockpit "glass") seemed to have little or no reaction to this foreign material. This led him to suppose that a small lens made out of the same material could probably be tolerated inside the human eye. Soon he began experimenting with plastic lens designs, and the modern era of intraocular lens implantation for cataract surgery was born.

About the same time that Ridley envisioned the plastic intraocular implant, José Barraquer in Columbia developed the idea of lamellar (layered) corneal surgery to alter the shape of the cornea. He discovered that lamellar keratoplasty could flatten the cone of a keratoconus patient, significantly reducing myopia.

In 1949 Barraquer described the principles of lamellar surgery. He changed the cornea's shape by removing the anterior cornea (the equivalent of today's corneal flap) with an instrument called a microkeratome, freezing it, and changing its shape with a mechanical lathe called the cryolathe. In the mid-1980s the cryolathe rose to its highest state of precision through automation. In 1985 Casimir Swinger developed a method of changing the shape of the cornea without freezing it. He did this using the microkeratome only. Then in 1987 Luis Ruiz, a protégé of Barraquer, modified the principles of microkeratome corneal resection (cutting) and used an automated form of the instrument to perform the operation in situ (directly on the eye). This procedure, called automated lamellar keratoplasty (ALK), was used to correct high levels of myopia and hyperopia.

Halfway around the globe, a handful of Russian ophthalmologists began research to determine whether or not RK (radial keratotomy, or straight-line incisions placed in a spoke-like pattern around the periphery of the cornea) could be effective if it was confined to the anterior side of the cornea. This would thereby avoid the long-term problems that arose from the disruption of the corneal endothelium in Sato's posterior keratotomies.

By the mid-1970s, Russian scientists such as Durney, Yenaleyev, and Fyodorov had determined that most of the radial keratotomy flattening effect could be obtained with sixteen or fewer incisions placed only on the anterior cornea. Fyodorov developed a system of anterior radial keratotomy that, by varying the number of incisions and the amount of uncut clear central zones between them, permitted him to carefully control the degree of visual correction. It was he who convinced the world that radial keratotomy (RK) could indeed reduce or eliminate myopia.

Radial keratotomy was introduced into the United States in 1978 by Leo Bores. It soon became a subject of great interest and careful scientific scrutiny. In 1980 the National Institutes of Health sponsored the PERK (Prospective Evaluation of Radial Keratotomy) study which provided factual, scientific data on radial keratotomy performed in a standard manner in nine centers across the United States.

The Arrival of the Excimer Laser

The first step in the evolution of laser surgery occurred when experts researched the application of laser technology to vision correction. In 1980 Beckman and Peyman and their associates used a carbon dioxide laser to create thermal shrinkage of the cornea in order to change corneal contour. A year later in 1981 John Taboada reported at a meeting of the

Aerospace Medical Association that the argon-fluoride excimer laser had the ability to indent eye tissue. Work then proceeded on ablation (microsurgical removal) of corneal tissue to flatten the cornea. Further evaluation was performed by Steve Trokel.

The first use of the excimer laser on blind human eyes took place in 1985 by Seiler in Germany. This was followed in 1987 in the United States. The procedure was called photorefractive keratectomy (PRK) and involved the ablation of the surface of the cornea to flatten its central portion in order to correct nearsightedness.

By 1990 and 1991, Pallikaris and Buratto and their associates had combined lamellar splitting (using the blade of a microkeratome to make a corneal flap, based on Barraquer's pioneering work forty years earlier) with excimer laser ablation of the exposed corneal bed. It was Pallikaris who coined the term LASIK (laser in-situ keratomileusis). This procedure took the moderately successful automated lamellar keratoplasty (ALK) procedure and added the incredible accuracy of the excimer laser to improve the results.

With LASIK, the realm of refractive surgery has been propelled into the space age dream of a nearly instantaneous, virtually discomfort free, refractive correction procedure, one that is literally sweeping the earth.

History Timeline of LASIK and Custom LASIK Surgery

- 1862 Topical eye anesthesia first used
- 1867 Keratometer developed measuring corneal Astigmatism.
- 1895 Faber performed first full thickness incision to correct astigmatism

- 1936 Sato of Japan did first radial keratotomies on back surface of cornea procedure, but later stopped due to poor results.
- 1948 Harold Ridley implanted first intraocular lens.
- 1949 José Barraquer of Columbia developed the first lamellar (layered) corneal surgery to alter the shape of the cornea. He used a micro-keratome to remove a flap tissue. He then froze it and changed the shape using a cryolathe. This lamellar surgery was an early forerunner to Lasik.
- 1970's Fyodorov et al developed radial keratotomy Soviet Union.
- 1978 Leo Bores performed first radial keratotomy in the United States.
- 1981 excimer laser developed
- 1985 micro-keratome refined by Swinger & Ruiz for lamellar surgery. ALK developed and performed immediate predecessor to LASIK.
- 1985 first excimer laser performed on human eye
- 1990 Pallikaris performs first LASIK procedure based on Barraquer work 40 years earlier.
- 1995 excimer laser approved by FDA in U.S. for low & moderate myopia
- 1997 excimer laser approved by FDA in U.S. for astigmatism
- 1998 excimer laser approved by FDA in U.S. for high myopia
- 1999 excimer laser approved by FDA in U.S. for farsightedness
- 2003 Custom Wavefront LASIK approved by FDA in U.S. for Custom LASIK procedures

Miraculous advances have taken place to help our patients achieve excellent vision. Custom LASIK is the culmination of innovation, technology, and scientific insight. The future holds promise for many patients who today can't be helped with Custom LASIK. The advances in vision correction will help those patients realize the dream of clear vision.

Made in United States
Troutdale, OR
11/03/2026

56852528R00066